A WOMAN DOCTOR'S GUIDE TO SKIN CARE

A WOMAN DOCTOR'S GUIDE TO SKIN CARE

Essential Facts and
Up-to-the-Minute Information on
Keeping Skin Healthy at Any Age

by

Wilma F. Bergfeld, M.D., F.A.C.P.

with

Shelagh Ryan Masline

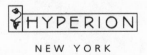

NEW YORK

LIBRARY OF CONGRESS CATALOGING-IN-PUBLICATION DATA
Bergfeld, Wilma F., 1938–
    A woman doctor's guide to skin care : essential facts and up-to-
the-minute information on keeping skin healthy at any age / Wilma
F. Bergfeld, with Shelagh Ryan Masline.
        p. cm.
    Includes bibliographical references and index.
    ISBN 0-7868-8100-3
    1. Skin—Care and hygiene. I. Masline, Shelagh A. R. II. Title.
RL87.B46 1995
616.5—dc20

                                                            95–1576
                                                            CIP

FIRST EDITION
10 9 8 7 6 5 4 3 2 1

To women who desire to know more about their skin
and how to keep it healthy

—Dr. Wilma F. Bergfeld

To the most important ladies in my life:
my daughter, Caitlin, and my mother, Eileen

—Shelagh Ryan Masline

ACKNOWLEDGMENTS

My thanks to the American Academy of Dermatology for their ten-year campaign to educate the public about the risks of sun exposure and skin cancer.

—Dr. Wilma F. Bergfeld

My thanks to Eileen Fallon and Laurie Abkemeier for their dedicated editorial and personal support.

—Shelagh Ryan Masline

CONTENTS

LIST OF ILLUSTRATIONS

A WOMAN DOCTOR'S GUIDE TO SKIN CARE

CHAPTER 1

The average woman's body is covered by eight pounds or seventeen square feet of skin. As the largest and one of the most important organs of your body, your skin acts as a barrier against the ravages of the environment—from the damaging ultraviolet rays of the sun to chemicals in makeup, smoke, and other pollutants in the air. Through its vast network of blood vessels and sweat glands, your skin also regulates your body's temperature and dispenses oxygen and nutrients to your nerves, glands, hair, and nails. It contains the sensory organs responsible for your sense of touch; it excretes waste through sweat glands; and exposure to the sun enables your body to create vitamin D, which is essential to good health. Yet your skin is delicate and often misunderstood or mistreated. Subject to the daily wear and tear of the environment, this vast organ suffers a barrage of insults from the outside.

The good news is that you have a great deal of control over the state of your skin, and in many ways you are the arbiter of your skin's fate. Gentle daily cleansing, for example, will wash away the residue of pollutants in the atmosphere; appropriate use of cosmetics tailored to your skin type will minimize the risk of negative reactions such as skin rashes; and taking advantage of the many combination skin care products available that include valuable sun protection will help slow down the aging effects of UV rays.

In this book we'll tell you how to take care of your skin, your most sizable and most visible organ. We'll also explore what can be done in the dermatologist's office, at the cosmetics counter of your department store, at your local drugstore, and in the privacy of your own bathroom, to keep your skin healthy and attractive. And, since your hair and nails are essentially extensions of your skin, we'll devote a special chapter to the basics of healthy hair and nail care.

GET TO KNOW THE FACTS

If you don't know the facts about your skin, you may be vulnerable to the misinformation, misrepresentation, and myths about skin care. False claims and rumors about skin crowd the pages of popular women's magazines. Let's begin by dismissing some of the more common myths:

MYTH: A light suntan can protect your skin.

FACT: A tan may protect you in the short run against sunburn, but it is no defense against wrinkling or skin cancer. *Any tan is an indication that skin damage has already taken place.* Someday that damage will show up in your skin in the form of premature aging—as age spots, wrinkles, and sagging skin—or possibly even skin cancer.

MYTH: Everyone needs a daily dose of sunshine to maintain good health.

FACT: Vitamin D, which is synthesized by sunlight, is necessary to help your body absorb calcium and phosphorus for healthy bones, teeth, and hair—but as little as ten to fifteen minutes of sun exposure each week helps your body make all the vitamin D you need.

Another fact to keep in mind is that most of us already get adequate amounts of vitamin D in our normal diet. Adults need 200 international units (IUs) a day, and children need 400 IUs. Fortified foods, such as dairy products and cereal, are good dietary sources of vitamin D. One cup of vitamin D–fortified milk, for example, contains 100 IUs.

And don't let the vitamin D myth prevent you from using sunscreen. A broad-based sunscreen is necessary to protect your skin from increased risk of cancer and premature aging.

MYTH: Everyone needs a moisturizer.

FACT: Teenagers who have oily skin are much better off without a moisturizer. However, most women over the age of twenty can benefit from using a moisturizer. If your skin feels tight and dry, or if you see wrinkles developing, you probably need one. A useful combination product, and one that is readily available today, is a moisturizer that also protects your skin from the sun.

MYTH: Applying extra moisturizer can help clear up dry and scaly patches on your skin.

FACT: Overmoisturizing is *not* the answer to all dry skin problems. Dry, flaky, or scaly patches on your face can be a sign of an allergic reaction or seborrheic dermatitis, and in these cases heavy moisturizers can worsen skin problems by clogging your pores. If your regular moisturizer is no longer effective, it's best to see your dermatologist to determine the underlying cause of your dry skin. Your dermatologist may recommend topical corticosteroids or anti-yeast medications.

MYTH: Everyone needs to use a toner or astringent.

FACT: Toners or astringents are great for people who have very oily or acne-prone skin, but they are not for everyone. For many people, especially those who already have dry skin, they can be too drying.

MYTH: Eating too much chocolate or fried foods causes acne.

FACT: Contrary to your parents' advice, acne is neither brought on nor made worse by eating foods like chocolate, ice cream, potato chips, or pizza. Foods that are greasy or fatty should be avoided for general health reasons, but not because they cause acne. You may be surprised to learn that it is actually foods that are high in iodine—such as iodized salt, shellfish, and seaweed—that can lead to outbreaks of acne.

MYTH: Exposure to sunlight can cure acne.

FACT: People who believe that a suntan can cure their acne are in for a rude awakening. A suntan is a very dangerous ruse, often employed by teenagers, to temporarily *conceal* acne. The long-term results are not worth it. Approximately one month after exposure to the sun, you will probably find yourself breaking out in whiteheads; this whitehead formation is linked to damage from ultraviolet rays and resultant clogging of pores.

MYTH: All surface skin disorders are stress-related.

FACT: It is true that many skin problems can be brought on or worsened by stress. But the fact is that stress is just one trigger of skin problems such as psoriasis and seborrhea. Your own genetic predisposition plays the most important role in determining whether or not you are prone to developing skin rashes. Other triggers of skin rashes include physical illness, overexposure to the sun, and cuts or scrapes.

MYTH: Expensive skin care products work best.

FACT: There is no evidence that the product you buy in an expensive department store is any better than the one available at your local drugstore. Unless you have a serious skin problem that requires the care of a dermatologist and prescription medicine, you don't have to spend a lot of money to take good care of your skin.

MYTH: Topical skin care products that contain collagen can make you look younger.

FACT: Most topical skin care products are made up of molecules far too large to penetrate the epidermis, let alone the inner dermis where collagen fibers are located. While collagen *injections* from your dermatologist can penetrate the dermis and smooth wrinkles by boosting the overall amount of collagen in your skin, collagen creams and lotions cannot. The most important products for most women's skin are mild cleansers, simple but effective moisturizers, and sunscreen (many cleansers and moisturizers already include sun protection).

MYTH: Hypoallergenic products are safe for anyone to use.

FACT: The tests used by cosmetic manufacturers are not regulated by any federal agency. A product advertised as hypoallergenic could have been tested on thousands of people, or just a few. There's no way of knowing. If you have sensitive skin, it's best to try out all new products—whether or not they are advertised as hypoallergenic—on a small patch of skin. If you experience no negative reaction (most notably a rash), gradually begin using the product more freely.

MYTH: Balding and hair loss are men's problems.

FACT: This is a common misconception. The fact is, if hair loss has been common on either side of your family, you may be genetically predisposed to shed hair at an early age. Thinning hair is a common problem that affects over 20 million women in the United States. The good news is that with the development of hair replacement products such as Minoxidil (available by prescription from your doctor), many women are now finding it possible to regrow their hair.

MYTH: If you're pregnant, you should probably postpone getting a perm.

FACT: Actually, this one is true. Pregnancy and nursing both have a major impact on your hormones, which can affect your hair and therefore the effectiveness of a perm. Women should also avoid having their hair colored during pregnancy—especially during the first trimester when your baby is developing major organs and is most vulnerable to harm. While there is no firm evidence that the chemicals in hair dye or perming products affect your baby, is it worth taking the chance?

CHAPTER 2

The skin is one of your body's most vital and complex organs, and healthy skin is as important to your overall well-being as are clear lungs and a sound heart. The skin is, after all, your body's number-one line of defense against physical injury and bacterial or chemical invasion.

In this chapter, we'll discuss the anatomy and structure of skin, and how it accomplishes important body functions. We'll also see how each layer of skin has a distinct set of characteristics and plays a unique role in protecting your body. And, since overall good health is the key to healthy skin, we'll introduce the concept of skin wellness. A healthy skin is the reflection of a healthy lifestyle. While some wrinkles are simply part of the natural aging process, many are due to actions completely under your control, such as overexposure to the sun or smoking cigarettes.

THE ANATOMY OF SKIN

Your skin is composed of two major layers: the *epidermis* and the *dermis*. The epidermis, or outermost layer of skin, produces proteins and keratin, which protect your body from harm-

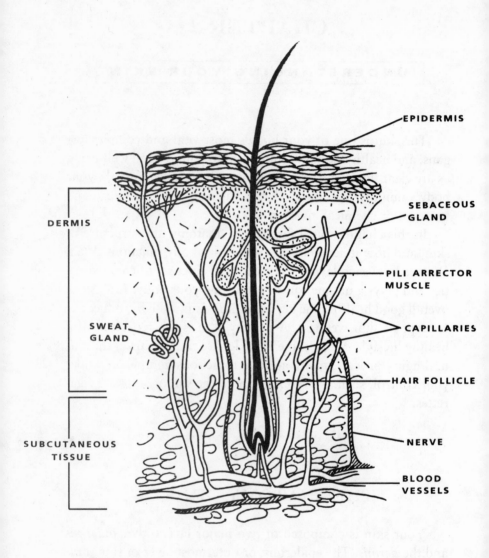

EPIDERMIS

DERMIS

SEBACEOUS
GLAND

PILI ARRECTOR
MUSCLE

CAPILLARIES

SWEAT
GLAND

HAIR FOLLICLE

SUBCUTANEOUS
TISSUE

NERVE

BLOOD
VESSELS

FIGURE 1 The Anatomy of Skin

ful environmental substances. The next layer of skin, the dermis, stores water and fat and helps regulate your body temperature. Connecting these two layers is the *basement membrane,* also known as the dermal/epidermal junction. Underlying both the dermis and the epidermis is *subcutaneous tissue,* which is primarily composed of fat and provides valuable insulation and calorie reserves. (See Figure 1, p. 8.)

THE EPIDERMIS

The primary function of the epidermis is to manufacture *keratin,* a tightly compacted protein that has immunological benefits and enables your skin to act as a waterproof barrier between you and the outside world. Keratin is the substance that protects your body from harmful environmental influences, such as cigarette smoke and pollutants. Melanin in the epidermis protects your skin from sunlight.

The epidermis is also a primary site of skin cell growth. At the bottom layer of the epidermis, *basal cells* grow, divide, and reproduce. New cells push mature cells upward, and as they travel they evolve into older, flatter *squamous cells.* When cells reach the top layer of the epidermis (the *stratum corneum*), they die and flake off. In this way, the cells of your skin constantly multiply, and your skin constantly renews and repairs itself in a controlled and orderly manner. (Turn to Chapter Four to read about uncontrolled cell growth, which can lead to skin cancer.)

The cells of your epidermis replace themselves approximately once every twenty-eight days. Cell turnover, of course, varies with age. A young woman may have new and glowing skin every two to three weeks, as dead skin cells are rapidly sloughed off and replaced. As we grow older, cell replacement slows, and the process doubles in length as we enter our sixties and seventies.

THE CELLS OF THE EPIDERMIS

The epidermis is composed of many different types of cells:

- **Squamous cells** lie in flat, scalelike profusion on the surface of your skin and are continuously shed as your skin renews itself.
- **Basal cells,** which are plump and round, are constantly being formed lower in the epidermis. They evolve into squamous cells as they rise to the skin's surface.
- **Melanocytes** reside deeper still in the epidermis and produce the pigment melanin. The amount of melanin in your skin accounts for variations in skin color. The more melanin you have in your skin, the darker your skin and the more resistant you are to the harmful ultraviolet rays of the sun.
- **Langerhans cells** make up only a small percentage of your epidermal cells, but are thought to play a valuable role in your body's immune system by helping the epidermis ward off outside infections and foreign materials. The langerhans cells have small tentacles, which reach out like small hands to sense and seize foreign substances; these cells then send dangerous substances to the lymph nodes where they are processed and dispelled from the body.

THE DERMIS

The dermis is responsible for a wide range of skin functions. This complex inner layer of skin contains a network of collagen and elastic fibers, lymph and blood vessels, sebaceous glands, nerve fibers, sweat glands, and hair follicles. Any time you injure yourself to the extent of drawing blood, you have injured your dermis and risk scarring.

Blood vessels and sweat glands in the dermis work together to regulate your body temperature. Nerve endings convey a wide range of sensations, from pain to pleasure, which travel all the way from the skin to the brain and back again. The dermis is also the determinant of many skin features, notably signs of the aging process. It is collagen and elastin in the dermis layer that give strength and elasticity to the skin, while sebaceous glands lubricate and soften the skin. As sun damage or age affects your dermis by decreasing collagen and elastic fibers, your skin may begin to wrinkle and sag.

THE ELEMENTS OF THE DERMIS

The dermis houses a number of different substances:

- **Blood vessels** in the dermis of your skin reach up to the epidermis to feed and nourish it. When blood circulation is stimulated, as in pregnancy, your skin becomes pink and rosy. As circulation through blood vessels in the skin slows—either with age or if you are a heavy smoker—your skin will become pale and sallow. Smoking causes blood vessels to constrict, reducing blood flow to the skin.
- **Collagen and elastic fibers** lend flexibility and strength to your skin. Wrinkling and sagging occur when these fibers are damaged or reduced by the sun or stretched with age.
- **Hair follicles** contain hair and act as an exit tract through which sebum and sweat reach the skin's surface.
- **Lymph vessels** in the dermis are part of the vast lymphatic system that produces, stores, and carries white blood cells throughout the body.
- **Nerve fibers** are responsible for our sense of touch.
- **Sebaceous glands** produce sebum, an oily substance that keeps your skin smooth and moist. Oversecretion of sebum, as in adolescence, exacerbates acne. As you grow older and the sebaceous glands slow production, dry skin and fine lines result.
- **Sweat glands** produce perspiration, which is secreted onto the skin surface; there it evaporates, cooling your skin and helping to regulate your body's temperature.
- The **pili arrector muscle** is the muscle attached to the hair follicle. When the muscle contracts, it produces "goose flesh."

THE BASEMENT MEMBRANE

Between the dermis and the epidermis is the basement membrane, a series of connecting tissues, which weaves the two layers together. The connection is extremely irregular, consisting of a number of fingerlike projections called *papillae*. Each papilla contains a network of collagen fibrils, blood vessels, and nerve endings. As skin ages, the basement membrane flattens, and there is a decrease in the amount and efficiency of the exchange of nutrients between the two layers.

SUBCUTANEOUS TISSUE

The subcutaneous tissue underlying the two major layers of skin contains sensory and motor nerves (like the dermis) that help account for our sense of touch. But, most important, fatty subcutaneous tissue functions as a kind of shock absorber. It gives the skin its flexibility and resilience, insulating your body and keeping the outside world from coming into direct contact with your bones. Subcutaneous tissue also acts as a storage site, absorbing chemicals, drugs, and nutrients.

SKIN WELLNESS

Skin wellness is an important part of our overall good health. Good health is part of healthy skin, and healthy skin mirrors a healthy lifestyle. Lifestyle choices such as a well-balanced diet and regular exercise not only contribute to your general well-being, they also reduce the level of stress in your day-to-day life and give your immune system a boost—accomplishments that in turn can add life and color to skin and decrease your susceptibility to many troublesome skin rashes.

What shape is *your* skin in? The answer to this question depends on a number of factors. To some extent your skin is affected by your own genetic makeup and changes over the years as you age. Yet your skin is also in large part an indication, both directly and indirectly, of your personal habits. A healthy skin is the reflection of the following important factors:

- Good skin care (which we will discuss later)
- A diet rich in fruits, vegetables, and fiber
- Regular exercise
- Consistent protection from the sun
- Control of stress
- Avoidance of unhealthy habits such as smoking, over-indulgence in alcohol, and drug abuse

MAINTAINING A WELL-BALANCED DIET

Your diet and lifestyle choices accumulate over the years and, along with built-in genetic factors, affect how your skin ages. But while you can't control your genes, you can do something about your diet.

A healthy diet is an essential part of your overall good health. A well-balanced diet can improve the color and texture of your skin and prevent nutrition-related skin disorders. To ensure that you maintain a healthy diet, follow these five important rules:

1. DRINK PLENTY OF FLUIDS

We should all drink at least eight glasses of water each day to cleanse our bodies of toxins and keep our body systems moving at peak efficiency. Water is an essential element of all metabolic processes and is especially important as we age.

2. CUT BACK ON FAT AND CALORIES

When you are young, it often seems like you can get away with eating just about anything. But a diet high in fat has long been linked to heart disease and certain forms of cancer. Current research also suggests that a high-fat diet may lead to skin cancer; researchers speculate that excess dietary fat may increase your risk of skin cancer by lowering your body's overall immune system function.

As you grow older, your body begins to lose muscle tissue, and, as a result, you burn fat and calories less efficiently. Your overall metabolism slows down, and you need to eat less to maintain a healthy weight. In order to compensate, try reducing the portion sizes of your favorite high-calorie and high-fat foods.

3. CHOOSE LOW-FAT DAIRY PRODUCTS

Dairy products such as low-fat or nonfat yogurt, cottage cheese, and skim milk are good choices when you want to reduce your fat intake without sacrificing calcium. Canned sardines and salmon are good nondairy sources of calcium. As a woman it's important that you continue to include calcium in your diet, even as you cut out fat and calories, in order to avoid osteoporosis in later life.

FAT: ANOTHER CAUSE OF SKIN CANCER?

A high-fat diet may also contribute to the development of skin cancer, according to the Baylor College of Medicine (Houston, Texas). In their recent two-year study of seventy-six skin cancer patients, half were put on a low-fat diet with 20 percent of calories from fat, and half consumed the average high-fat diet of 40 percent of calories from fat. Findings revealed that low-fat dieters developed an average of only three additional precancerous tumors over that time, while those on the high-fat diet developed an average of ten. The experts concluded that excess fat in the diet may increase your risk of skin cancer by lowering your body's overall immune system function.

4. EAT NUTRIENT-RICH FRUITS AND VEGETABLES

As you eliminate high-calorie foods loaded with fats and sugar, add plenty of fruits and vegetables to your diet. Foods such as broccoli, sweet potatoes, carrots, nectarines, and citrus fruits are packed with vitamins, minerals, and fiber.

5. INCREASE YOUR FIBER INTAKE

Try to get your fiber intake up to at least 25 grams per day. Whole grains, bran cereals, brown rice, beans, and lentils are good sources of fiber, as are fresh fruits and vegetables.

GET REGULAR EXERCISE

Exercise makes you look and feel better. As well as improving overall posture and muscle tone, regular exercise puts color in your cheeks. After a workout, your skin takes on a special healthy glow. Aerobic exercise increases blood circulation, enhancing the flow of oxygen and nutrients throughout your body, including your skin. An added benefit of exercise is that it is a natural way to relieve stress. As you age, exercise is increasingly necessary to burn off fat and tone muscles.

PROTECT YOUR SKIN WHILE YOU EXERCISE

While exercise is an indisputable plus for your skin, certain precautions should be taken. Exposure to the sun is a constant concern if you exercise outdoors. For the greatest protection, dermatologists recommend that you apply a waterproof, broad spectrum sunscreen with an SPF (Sun Protection Factor) of at least 15 on a daily basis.

Certain skin ailments are also associated with exercise. Sweat is the greatest culprit: It makes your body more vulnerable to invasion of the fungi that live on your skin. In fact, many infectious microbes live on the skin all the time, waiting for a break in the skin surface or help from heat and perspiration to multiply and cause rashes and infections.

The solution? Don't quit exercising! Simply incorporate appropriate clothing and protection into your exercise regime. Try some of the following measures:

- Always wear sunscreen when exercising outdoors.
- Protect your skin with moisturizer before swimming in a chlorinated pool.
- Protect your skin with a moisturizing sunscreen in cold and windy conditions.
- Wear loose clothing when you play softball or go for a run.
- Choose fabrics, such as cotton, that let skin breathe.
- Use a gentle, nonirritating soap to wash workout clothes.
- Remove makeup and jewelry before working out.
- Wear kneepads and elbowpads when in-line skating.

EXERCISE-RELATED SKIN PROBLEMS

Exercise is beneficial to your whole body, including your skin. But skin problems are often an inadvertent side effect of exercise:

- **Blisters** Blisters occur when repeated friction or pressure causes the epidermis to separate from the dermis, creating a painful pocket that gradually fills with fluid. Runners who suffer from blisters should be sure to wear shoes that fit properly. Small blisters respond to self-treatment with Band-Aids. Your dermatologist may have to drain very large blisters, and apply a topical antibiotic to prevent secondary infection.
- **Bunions** A bunion is a painful inflammation of the skin that is caused by constant friction and pressure. Bunions most commonly occur at the base of the big

toe and are caused by wearing shoes that fit poorly. You may also have a genetic predisposition to bunions, which run in families. Like the other disorders described here, bunions are common in, but not unique to, athletes. Anyone who wears shoes that do not fit properly is vulnerable to foot problems. Most bunions can be successfully treated with heat and moisture, but serious bunions may have to be removed by your orthopedist or podiatrist.

- **Corns** Corns, or cone-shaped bumps that result from the hardening of the outer layer of skin, are caused by constant friction or pressure. Wearing shoes that fit properly is the best way to prevent corns. Over-the-counter corn pads can provide immediate relief from the pain, while large corns may have to be trimmed by your dermatologist.

- **Calluses** Calluses are thickened areas of skin that are due to constant friction or pressure. Your body develops calluses as a defensive measure to eliminate the possibility of damage to the soft skin beneath them. The hands and feet are the most common areas of occurrence; writer's bump, for instance, is a callus that develops on the side of the finger due to constant pressure. Calluses can be softened by applying warm, moist compresses. Your best bet, however, is to eliminate the underlying cause of calluses.

- **Excessive Sweating and Smelling** It's a fact of life: When you exercise, you work up a sweat. Sweating is how your body regulates its temperature while you exercise, whereas odor is caused by the interaction of perspiration with the bacteria that live on your skin. Yet as natural as they may be, excessive sweating and smelling can also be embarrassing.

  Antimicrobial underarm deodorants and more powerful antiperspirants, which contain chemicals that block sweating, control perspiration and odor in most people. But if you suffer from excessive sweating to an unusual degree—even when you don't exercise—you may have a medical condition known as *hyperhidrosis*. Your dermatologist can prescribe stronger antiperspirants for this condition.

- **Jogger's Nipples** Inflamed, itchy, and sensitive jogger's nipples are the result of constant friction across the skin from your T-shirt or bra. Physical barriers such as sports bras, Band-Aids, or dressings can prevent the problem. If the problem is severe, your dermatologist may prescribe topical corticosteroids.

- **Rough Skin** Rough skin on the heels of runners is usually caused by friction with shoes. In fact, anyone who wears shoes that do not fit well can develop rough skin. To eliminate rough skin, gently rub with a pumice stone after bathing. Applying moisturizer will also help.

PROTECT YOURSELF FROM THE SUN

Exposure to sunlight over time and periodic episodes of overexposure to sunlight—especially when they lead to sunburn and blistering—are the causes of at least 90 percent of all skin cancers. Yet each summer the beaches are crowded with sun worshipers in pursuit of the perfect tan. The fact is that a tan should no longer be looked upon as glamorous, attractive, or healthy in any way. It's time to realize that getting a tan affects your skin in much the same way smoking a cigarette affects your lungs. Sun damage occurs with every unprotected sun exposure and accumulates over the course of a lifetime. To protect your skin from sun damage, try to avoid midday exposure and apply sunscreen whenever you go outside.

CONTROL STRESS

Whenever your body perceives stress—whether you are late for work, or when the pilot on an airplane tells you to tighten your seatbelt because there's turbulence ahead—your body kicks in with its famous "fight or flight" hormones. These stress hormones are released by your brain to help you cope with the difficult situation at hand.

Yet beyond managing the stress itself, a multitude of skin disorders are triggered or worsened by stress. A job interview, for example, can make you break out into a sweat and consequently create or aggravate a rash. Acne, hives, eczema, psoriasis, and seborrhea are among the many skin conditions that are influenced by stress.

There are schools of thought that say a little stress is good for you; for example, stress might motivate you to get out of bed earlier so you can make it to work on time. But the most damaging stressful situations are those that we cannot control—such as when the plane is "experiencing turbulence." Actually *we* are experiencing the turbulence. Fortunately, there are many ways we can deal with stress in special situations and in our day-to-day lives.

POPULAR STRESS-BUSTERS

Following is a list of stress-busters, ranging from the esoteric to the mundane. The list is by no means conclusive. Engaging in a favorite hobby—whether it is knitting or woodworking—is often the best way for an individual to relieve stress. But you may also want to try:

- Daily exercise
- A post-exercise visit to the sauna, steam room, or whirlpool
- Massage

- Meditation
- Yoga
- Biofeedback
- Visualization
- Taking a nap
- Reading a book
- Watching a movie

AVOID BAD HABITS

An old adage has it that "your skin never forgets." If you stay out late and don't get enough sleep, for example, you may end up with dark shadows under your eyes. If you engage in more serious bad habits—most commonly, smoking cigarettes or the abuse of alcohol or drugs—the consequences to your health, and the impact on your skin, are also more serious.

Chronic smoking over a period of years leads to an unattractive condition with a name to match it: "smoker's face." As well as leading to serious health problems such as high blood pressure and liver disease, a few too many drinks on a regular basis can cause broken capillaries in your face and misshapen features, such as a bulbous nose. And drug abuse not only destroys your health, it also leaves its mark on your skin. In other words, when you engage in self-destructive behavior, you are abusing your whole body, including your skin.

SMOKING

Smoking causes lung cancer, heart disease, emphysema—and "smoker's face." Over time, nicotine constricts the blood vessels that carry nutrients to the surface of the skin, gradually turning the skin color of chronic smokers pale and sallow. Additional wrinkles, creases, and lines eventually surround the lips and eyes of smokers. Cigarette smoking also slows th skin after surgery.

If you are a smoker and you care about your sk consider quitting. The American Cancer Society and the local chapters of the American Lung and American Heart Associations have books, videos, and group programs to help you quit for good. If you are a nonsmoker, make sure that your rights to smoke-free spaces are upheld.

ALCOHOL

Like smoking, drinking has an impact on your looks as well as your health. If you regularly have more than one or two alcoholic drinks a day, you may have a drinking problem. Many people's faces flush after they've had several drinks; this is due to dilation of the tiny blood vessels in the skin of your face and neck. Over time, these blood vessels lose their ability to constrict. This results in a chronic alcoholic flush in which a network of broken spider veins may appear and spread across the drinker's nose and cheeks. If you continue drinking, these veins may become increasingly swollen and disfiguring.

DRUGS

When prescribed or recommended by your doctor, drugs can be a great help in relieving various symptoms and ailments. Drug abuse, on the other hand, can damage your overall health and can also have a negative impact on your skin.

Different drugs leave different marks on your skin. Smoking marijuana, for example, can lead to acne flare-ups and hives. Tranquilizers and stimulants have both been known to cause allergic reactions.

Snorting cocaine is associated with extremely dry mouth and lips. Over time, the use of cocaine can severely damage nasal blood vessels, mucous membranes, and cartilage. Eventually, many people who snort cocaine may actually create a hole between the nostrils. At this level of drug abuse, surgical intervention is necessary.

Clearly drug abuse—like smoking and alcoholism—has severe consequences for your health and can physically as well as cosmetically damage your skin. If you haven't engaged in these negative forms of behavior, don't start. If you already have a problem, get help before it's too late.

CARING FOR YOUR SKIN AS YOU AGE

The healthy skin care habits that we have described in this chapter can be yours for a lifetime. In fact, the more care you lavish on your skin, the better you will age. And, as you will see in the next chapter, good skin is not just for the young. Healthy skin is possible at any age.

CHAPTER 3

Until recently, scientists believed that aging skin was simply an inexorable process of deterioration, firmly etched into our genes. A little sagging or drooping here, a wrinkle there, a few brown age spots—all these uncomfortable developments were regarded as part of the normal aging process, destined to begin as early as our twenties or thirties. But no more!

Today, dermatologists stress that the major cause of skin aging is our cumulative exposure to the sun. While the luck of the draw—in this case, genetics—plays an important part in who has the finest skin, the habits of a lifetime usually play an even greater role in how your skin ages.

In addition to the personal choices you make to control the shape your skin is in, today it is possible to slow the aging process and even reverse it in many cases. Scientists have developed breakthrough treatments that can take years off the way you look. In an effort to turn back the clock, women are increasingly turning to products such as alpha hydroxy acids and Retin-A, as well as procedures including collagen injections and chemical peels. In this chapter, we'll take a look at how skin ages, and offer positive suggestions to help keep your skin youthful and healthy.

HOW YOUR SKIN AGES

Dermatologists note that there are actually two ways in which your skin ages: through the natural aging process and through photoaging. And more and more experts today agree that the majority of deep wrinkles and furrows on our faces are not just part of this so-called normal aging process—in fact, they are directly attributable to photoaging (damage due to exposure to the sun).

This is the crucial difference between normal chronological aging and photoaging: While you do have a measure of control over chronological aging—through healthy habits or dermatological interventions—you have virtually 100 percent power over the effects of photoaging. (No one forces you to bask for hours on the beach without the benefit of appropriate protection.)

You may think it's normal to have wrinkles appear on your face by age thirty-five or so, but dermatologists disagree. The majority of fine lines and wrinkles at this time are due to your previous exposure to damaging ultraviolet rays from the sun over the course of your lifetime. Our skin would remain smooth and firm for years longer if we exercised more effective sun protection.

NORMAL AGING VS. PHOTOAGING

As skin ages, the rate of cell production slows, gradually causing cell turnover and cell repair to become less effective. More and more water is also lost, which leads to drying and cracking and decreases your skin's ability to act as a protective barrier. Skin tone may grow sallow as pigment-producing cells slow in activity.

The normal aging process of your skin gradually leads to thinner skin, increased dryness, fine wrinkles, excess facial hair, and changes in facial contour. Skin goes through a series of changes as we pass through each decade of our lives, and we will examine those changes—and what to do about them—in this chapter.

In contrast, sun-exposed skin becomes permanently thickened. To get an idea of how your skin would age if you did not constantly expose it to the sun, take a look at the parts of your body that receive the least ultraviolet exposure, such as the smooth skin of your buttocks. There will probably be little if any dryness or roughness—and even if there is, it will be far less severe than on the sun-exposed areas of your body.

According to the American Academy of Dermatology, exposure to the sun is responsible for the majority of wrinkles and age spots on a mature face. In fact, up to 80 percent of what is considered normal aging is actually photoaging. Even more serious, long-term exposure to the sun damages your skin's basic structure, leading to premature aging, benign skin tumors, and increasing your risk of skin cancer.

Photoaging involves damage to the dermis caused by the long ultraviolet rays of the sun. These extensive wavelengths penetrate deeply into the layers of your skin, causing abnormalities in the proteins that ordinarily keep your skin flexible and resilient. The cosmetic result is sagging, wrinkled, and unevenly colored skin; the medical result is an increased risk of skin cancer.

PROTECT YOUR SKIN FROM THE RAVAGES OF THE SUN

The fact is, the best things you can do for your skin are either free or yours for the price of a sunscreen:

* Avoid exposure to the sun between the hours of 10 A.M. and 3 P.M.
* Use a broad-based sunscreen with an SPF of at least 15 *every day*—even when it's cloudy.
* Wear a broad-brimmed hat and protective clothing to guard your skin from the sun.

THE STAGES AND AGES OF YOUR SKIN

Your skin passes through a multitude of stages as you grow older. While there is a great deal of overlapping, and every woman's skin is unique, there are certain sets of characteristics generally shared by each decade—from the overactive glands and hormones that lead to acne in teenagers, to the first appearances of fine lines and the increasing need for moisturizers in our thirties, to the loss of estrogen-dependent collagen and skin elasticity after menopause.

Fortunately, a wide variety of natural, cosmetic, and dermatological procedures are available to counteract or slow many of the less than pleasant aspects of the skin's aging process. In this section, we'll trace our skin through the decades and explore some of the natural and cosmetic ways to cope with the many changes that take place over time. Then we'll look at the newest and most sophisticated dermatological techniques— some of which can quite literally peel away years from your skin.

ADOLESCENCE

Apart from a skinned knee or the occasional case of poison ivy, young children tend to have few skin problems. But when hormones kick in during adolescence, the skin, along with the rest of the body, is in for an exciting period of change. Stretch marks may appear in young women for the first time, as their new adult bodies begin to expand and take shape. And during this time, the body dramatically steps up production of *androgens,* the hormones that cause sebaceous glands in the skin to expand and produce excess oil. *Acne* is a sign of androgen excess. (Hair loss, hirsutism, and obesity are other conditions associated with androgen excess.)

The key to avoiding acne is to keep facial and scalp oil control. It's best to cleanse the skin with a mild soap twice during this time. Moisturizers, on the other hand, are not only unnecessary for the vast majority of teenagers, they may actually clog pores and complicate acne. Washing your hair on a daily basis will also help keep scalp oil under control and decrease your risk of acne (since oil on your hair will often find its way to your face).

Whatever your age, healthy skin is also, of course, the reflection of a healthy lifestyle and a positive attitude. Some teenagers indulge in fad diets, which can be reflected in their complexions. Pale skin, for example, may be a sign of an eating disorder such as anorexia or bulimia. Still, for many healthy, active teens, these years can be very good ones for the skin. Teenagers who follow a balanced diet and engage in regular exercise will be rewarded with good muscle tone and circulation, a big plus for healthy skin. Exercise will also help decrease the stress known to accompany the adolescent years. In addition, it's important to steer clear of bad habits such as smoking and drinking, temptations that begin to rear their ugly heads during this decade. Likewise, teens should remember to exercise good "sun sense"; the first twenty years of life are those in which we typically experience up to 80 percent of our lifetime exposure to—and subsequent damage from—the sun.

Acne: The Teenage Plague

Although acne can occur at any age, it is a common affliction among teenagers. As teenagers mature sexually, hormonal changes stimulate the sebaceous glands in the hair follicles of the skin. Instead of providing a normal amount of sebum, the fatty acid that lubricates your skin, sebaceous glands begin working overtime. The follicles become clogged with sebum, and bacteria multiply in blocked channels. The result is acne, inflamed and swollen blemishes that are often filled with pus.

The main treatment of acne consists of good personal hygiene and following your dermatologist's advice about the treatment of blemishes. If your acne is severe, your doctor may prescribe topical medications and/or oral antibiotics to keep it under control.

THE TWENTIES

Most women enter their twenties with a sigh of relief. Skin is clear, pores are tight, and coloring is even. Many women will not even require a moisturizer until their thirties, while those who never had especially oily skin may want to lightly moisturize now due to decreased activity of the sebaceous glands. Simple skin cleansing, good sun protection, a well-balanced diet, and a sensible exercise program are all that's needed to add up to healthy skin for most women in their twenties.

For those of you still experiencing persistent acne, it may be linked to hormonal activity—especially if the flare-ups occur during the week prior to your menstrual period. This will likely continue throughout your childbearing years. Birth control pills also have a powerful impact on hormonal activity, and may contribute to acne problems.

PREGNANCY AND YOUR SKIN

Pregnant women have a special glow, so they say, and there is actually some physiological basis to this maxim. In addition to the influence of joyful anticipation, a pregnant woman experiences a major increase in the amount of blood in circulation necessary to support her fetus. And this usually brings a natural rosiness to the skin's surface.

Of course, as most women are well aware, pregnancy also brings its share of difficulties. It is without a doubt a period of profound hormonal, physiological, and emotional change in a woman's life.

Hyperpigmentation

Hyperpigmentation, or the darkening of certain skin areas, is thought to take place due to heightened hormonal stimulation. It is most evident in dark-skinned and dark-haired women, and the areas that may be affected include the nipples, vulva, anus, and inner thighs. Freckles and birthmarks may also darken during pregnancy. While any suspicious changes in a mole should be brought to the attention of your dermatologist, most of these changes are harmless and largely diminish after you give birth.

Melasma

Melasma, or "the mask of pregnancy," is a darkening of pigmentation on facial skin, another condition due to the massive hormonal changes taking place in your body at this time. Exposure to the sun and genetic factors may also play a role in melasma. Skin usually returns to its normal color over the course of the year following birth.

Skin Tags

Skin tags are harmless growths that often alarm women during pregnancy. Also known as papillomas, skin tags are fine stalks of flesh-colored or slightly pigmented skin growths that are commonly found on the necks of pregnant women. They may also develop on the chest, under the breasts, on the inner thighs, or on the face. Removal of skin tags is usually deferred until after women give birth. Your dermatologist can then remove small ones with a special scissors. Broader skin tags may require removal by electrosurgery or cryosurgery.

Spider Veins, Purpura, and Angiomas

The increase in the amount of blood circulating through the body can contribute to blood vessel problems, such as *spider*

veins, black and blue marks known as *purpura,* and *angiomas.*
Spider veins are harmless broken blood vessels, which many
women develop with age regardless of pregnancy. If they bother
you, they can be removed by your dermatologist after pregnancy. In the final trimester, extra stress on capillaries can cause
women to bruise more easily; this bruising, or purpura, usually
clears up soon after birth. Angiomas are small blood vessel tumors known as cherries. After pregnancy they often fade, or
they can be removed through electrodessication.

Stretch Marks

Among the many skin changes that can be expected during
pregnancy are the very well-known stretch marks, which are due
to tearing of collagen and elastin fibers when rapid weight gain
takes place. Massaging stretch marks with a moisturizer may
help, and over time they will fade and become less noticeable.

Varicose Veins and Hemorrhoids

Varicose veins, which appear in more than 40 percent of
pregnant women, can pose a major problem during pregnancy.
So can painful *hemorrhoids,* which are varicose veins in the anal
region. These conditions are thought to result from a combination of factors during pregnancy, particularly increased blood
flow and relaxed blood vessel walls. More blood flowing
through weakened vein walls will cause backup pressure and
swelling.

There seems to be a hereditary component in varicose veins;
if your mother had them when she was pregnant, you probably
will too. The best ways to cope with varicose veins and hemorrhoids during pregnancy are:

- Avoid excessive weight gain.
- Continue to exercise sensibly during pregnancy.
- Periodically elevate your feet and try to sleep on your
  side, to promote blood flow and minimize pressure
  on blood vessels.

- Avoid wearing constrictive clothing.
- Wear support hose.

While most swollen veins shrink after delivery, in some cases they become a progressive problem. Treatments range from covering with makeup to destruction by electrosurgery, laser therapy, vein stripping, and sclerotherapy.

THE THIRTIES

The good news is that your skin can still be attractively taut and smooth in your thirties. With good genes and effective sun protection, you may be able to reach the age of thirty-five without a wrinkle or a spot. Keeping your weight down and getting all the sleep you need are also helpful.

Still, small changes begin to take place in this decade. The delicate skin under your eyes is beginning to thin. While you may have been able to pull an all-nighter in your twenties and be none the worse for wear, a night out at the clubs in your thirties may generate puffy dark circles under your eyes. These are due to increased fat and sluggish blood flow.

Your skin is also less elastic than it was in your teens and twenties, and the first faint lines may begin to appear on your face. Very often these are the laugh lines around your mouth.

SKIN TIPS

- To hide dark circles under your eyes, consider using a concealer one shade lighter than your natural skin tone.
- To cure puffy eyes, apply cool water and ice. Wet tea bags may also reduce swelling.

If you haven't already launched your personal skin protection program, now is the time. Healthy skin for the thirtysomething woman usually begins with the daily application of a moisturizer that also contains a Sun Protection Factor of at least 15. Almost all moisturizers today offer sun protection, so it's easiest to get sun protection and moisture in one product. Wear the product every day—because ultraviolet rays of the sun are present all day long, all year long. On especially sunny days, you may also want to wear a broad-brimmed hat or visor.

Save Face: Quit Smoking

While smoking has been definitively linked to many serious and potentially fatal forms of cancer, heart disease, and emphysema, the harmful effects of smoking on your skin are not as well known. But if you're in your thirties and you're still smoking, you may eventually be forced to confront in your mirror the unpleasant reflection of "smoker's face," yet one more hazard of this dangerous addiction. Nicotine is believed to cause constriction of the blood vessels that carry nutrients to the surface of the skin, causing the skin color of chronic smokers to appear pale and sallow. Wrinkles, creases, and lines come to surround the smokers' lips (in pucker lines) and eyes (in crow's-feet). Cigarette smoking can also slow the healing of wounds after surgery, including plastic surgery (most likely due to poor capillary circulation in the skin as the result of smoking).

No one pretends that quitting smoking is easy. Yet today there are a number of self-help and group programs that can help you withdraw from this destructive and life-threatening habit. Nicotine gum and patches are also available by prescription from your physician to help ease withdrawal from the powerful addictive influence of nicotine. Additional information on the effects of smoking and how to quit are available from the American Cancer Society or the local chapters of the American Lung and American Heart associations (See Appendix I: Resources, p. 175).

THE FORTIES

As you enter your forties, your hide gets tougher. Skin tone and texture have begun to undergo serious changes. Your facial tone is duller, and your skin is less supple. Your skin is no longer as tight as it used to be; pores on the cheeks, and especially on the nose, will appear larger than they used to.

There's at least a 50 percent probability that you'll develop one or two age or liver spots in this decade. These flat, brown marks may appear on your face, hands, back, or feet, and are a result of cumulative exposure to sunlight over the years. On your legs, patterns of thin, red spider veins may be emerging.

Women have to be particularly careful to avoid the insidious weight gain that starts to occur in the late thirties and early forties. Diet and exercise are especially important at this time. Weight gain can lead to any number of health and cosmetic problems, from obesity to sagging skin. Cellulite, those distinctive dimples of fat, may appear on your thighs and buttocks when you reach your forties, especially if you are overweight.

Overall, the forties are when time really begins to catch up with you. Deep furrows on the forehead may be joined by crow's-feet around the eyes and laugh or frown lines around the mouth and nose. Circles under the eyes may grow into pouches; and speaking of pouches, if you've put on a few pounds, you may also develop a little fat deposit under your chin. Even if you've led a healthy lifestyle—and your skin continues to hold up just fine—maintenance will require an increasing amount of effort on your part.

THE INCREASING NEED FOR MOISTURE IN MIDDLE AGE

The bottom line is that dry skin is the cause of many of these problems. This is because sweat glands grow smaller and less effective as we age. The liberal use of moisturizer can happily counteract many of the skin problems associated with aging. So the first rule is, don't stint with the moisturizer: Slather it on.

- Cleanse your face and body with a soap that has moisturizer in it.
- Pour moisturizing gel into your bath or on a washcloth when you shower.
- Use a washcloth or loofah in your bath or shower to slough off dead skin cells and restore a glow to dull skin.
- Hydrate before moisturizing. While your skin is still damp, apply moisturizer over your entire body, paying special attention to your face. Damp skin can hold more moisture.

If you haven't done so already, in your forties you may begin to explore the vast array of antiaging products at your fingertips. Many skin care companies, for example, advertise overnight replenishing creams; these are heavier moisturizing creams than the light ones you will continue to use during the day.

The hottest new antiaging alternatives are prescription Retin-A and over-the-counter alpha hydroxy acids (AHAs). AHAs are fruit- and milk-based preparations that may help even out skin contours and soften fine lines. They should be applied every morning after cleansing with a mild soap and before applying sunscreen.

THE FIFTIES AND SIXTIES

By now your skin is acquiring true character. Fine wrinkles and laugh lines may deepen into folds in your fifties and sixties. In addition to wrinkling, skin can begin to droop and sag, and some women may begin to develop a jowly appearance.

Skin tone is also likely to become increasingly uneven in your fifties. Overall, everyone's skin grows lighter with age, due to decreased circulation—but those of us who have been exposed to the sun over the years may be developing an increasing number of age or liver spots. Most *solar lentigines,* the dermatological term for these harmless but cosmetically unappealing marks, can be covered up with a concealer. You can also explore the alternative of Retin-A with your dermatologist. Over time, the application of Retin-A, which is available by prescription only, can help smooth wrinkles and fade age spots.

Many of the changes taking place in skin at this time are part of the normal aging process, in which supportive collagen and elastin simply grow thinner over time. This is especially true for postmenopausal women because a woman's skin derives so much moisture and fullness from estrogen-dependent collagen.

After menopause when estrogen is no longer produced, moisturizing must become an even more important part of your regular skin care routine. Many postmenopausal women take hormone replacement therapy (HRT) to prevent osteoporosis. An added benefit of HRT is that skin remains moister and fuller. However, HRT has many risks as well as benefits and should be thoroughly discussed with your gynecologist.

In the long run, whether due to good genes or bone structure, some people simply age better than others. But it's always important to keep in mind that lifestyle plays a pivotal part in how you age. Taking good care of yourself in general will help your skin age as gracefully as possible, along with the rest of your body.

HOW TO LOOK YOUNGER

The ever increasing number of antiaging products and procedures are probably the hottest topics in skin care today. Everyone, it seems, wants to turn back—or at least slow down—the ticks of their own personal aging clocks. Consequently, there is a plethora of new antiaging products making a variety of promises to renew and revitalize your skin, or simply to make you look ten years younger. Topical products include alpha hydroxy acids and Retin-A; and chemical peels, dermabrasion, collagen and fat injections, face lifts, neck lifts, and liposuction are among the many antiaging procedures performed by dermatologists and plastic surgeons. Although none of these products or procedures work miracles, some do indeed give the temporary appearance of younger-looking skin.

PRESCRIPTION FOR YOUNGER SKIN

No discussion of antiaging would be complete without a discussion of the two hottest skin care products on the market today: alpha hydroxy acids and Retin-A. While both may have uncomfortable side effects, each seems to have valid antiaging qualities as well. No serious medical problems have been associated with the use of alpha hydroxy acids or Retin-A, although both have been known to cause temporary skin irritation and redness. While the FDA is monitoring the use of AHAs and Retin-A, neither drug is FDA-approved as an antiaging product.

Alpha Hydroxy Acids (AHAs)

Smooth and penetrating, alpha hydroxy acids act as exfoliators and moisturizers. Regular use of AHAs may counteract some of the effects of aging, by smoothing fine lines and improving skin tone. The strength of AHAs is dependent on their acid concentration.

The most common alpha hydroxy acids are glycolic acid (often a product of sugarcane); lactic acid (which may be extracted from sour milk); and pyruvic acid (commonly derived from apples). Over-the-counter AHAs contain 3 to 8 percent acid; more powerful prescription products may include some 8 to 40 percent acid. All of these acids are basically skin exfoliators. They appear to work by breaking the bond that holds cells together, thereby enabling your body to slough off dead skin cells and speed up cell renewal.

While many dermatologists recommend AHAs to soften rough skin and erase fine lines, the Food and Drug Administration (FDA) has yet to decide on whether or not these products actually deliver on their promises. But there do appear to be some hopeful signs.

Retin-A

Retin-A, or retinoic acid, is a vitamin A derivative that has long been used to treat acne. Known medically as tretinoin, Retin-A acts as an exfoliator. In 1988, an editorial in the *Journal of the American Medical Association* sent age-conscious consumers rushing out to their dermatologists. The news was out that Retin-A could soften and alleviate wrinkling of the skin.

While Retin-A may not be precisely the fountain of youth imagined by early enthusiasts, over time it *can* make skin more uniform in texture and color, make brown spots disappear, and soften fine lines. All this, however, comes at a price. Retin-A may cause unpleasant side effects, such as red and/or dry skin. Moreover, because it is for cosmetic, not medical, purposes, its cost is not covered by most insurance.

Still, many women swear by Retin-A. Today this drug, which is available by prescription only, is recommended by dermatologists on a regular basis to counteract the effects of aging. Although Retin-A has not been approved as a wrinkle treatment, doctors are permitted to use FDA-approved prescription drugs in any medical way they wish.

The most common forms of Retin-A are creams and gels. The product comes in various concentrations, but even low concentrations of the drug may leave skin temporarily dry, scaly, and red. Retin-A should be used only under the guidance of a trained and experienced dermatologist.

NEW NONSURGICAL TECHNIQUES FOR A YOUNGER SKIN

There was a time when a surgical face-lift was the only way to rid your skin of fine lines and wrinkles. Today there are a number of alternatives. In addition to the skin care products mentioned above, a variety of nonsurgical procedures is available that can help you look younger without experiencing the risks of surgery. These techniques can counteract to some extent the effects of the natural aging process, the impact of facial expressions over the years, and cumulative exposure to the sun. Most of these procedures are done under local anesthesia in the dermatologist's office.

Nonsurgical cosmetic treatments—including *chemical peels, dermabrasion, collagen* and *fat injections,* and *liposuction*—have so far proved most appealing to women in their thirties and forties who want to improve their appearance, but do not yet desire or require a face-lift. These treatments may in addition be more effective in this age group, since the skin remains more elastic and responsive in younger women. Since these procedures are relatively new, expensive, and controversial, it's important to choose the right dermatologist—one who is both certified and trained, and also someone to whom you can speak directly and openly about your own personal goals and concerns.

Chemical Peels

A chemical peel repairs uneven pigment and sun damage, and eliminates fine lines by actually peeling away the top layers of the skin. This procedure is basically a controlled wound, in which mild acid works to burn off surface layers of skin. A chemical peel can eliminate brown spots and actinic keratoses (precancerous conditions of rough, red or brown, scaly patches on the skin). And, in addition to evening out overall skin tone, a chemical peel can smooth out crow's-feet around the eyes and fine lines around the mouth.

There are three types of chemical peels: superficial, medium, and deep. Your dermatologist can help you decide which, if any, is right for you. Middle-aged women with light complexions and light eyes are the best candidates for chemical peels; olive-skinned women with dark eyes face a greater risk of complications, such as scars and dark spots. Medium and deep peels are painful and complicated procedures, and while a light peel has fewer side effects, you may still experience swelling, redness, and extreme sensitivity to the sun.

Dermabrasion

Dermabrasion is a procedure similar to the chemical peel, but instead of an acid, a hand-held, high-speed rotary wheel is used to remove the epidermis, or top layer of skin. Whereas a chemical peel is generally used to treat fine wrinkles, dermabrasion is an effective treatment for deeper imperfections, such as smooth scars left by acne, accidents, or previous surgery. Dermabrasion is also preferable to a chemical peel for people with darker skin since it is less likely to produce side effects such as changes in skin color.

Collagen Injections

Injecting purified bovine collagen into wrinkles is yet another way to make them disappear—at least temporarily. The procedure works on large wrinkles, deep furrows, creases between the mouth and nose, and furrows on your forehead, by plumping them up with collagen. The number of collagen injections required depends upon the depth of the wrinkles. The effects last between three and nine months. Side effects can include temporary bruising, redness, and swelling.

Some concerns about collagen persist. If you have an immunological disorder, collagen injections are not a good idea. In addition, a small percentage of the population is allergic to bovine collagen, and the FDA is continuing to study whether collagen is linked to connective tissue disorders.

Fat Injections

Fat injections are another technique to fill in unwanted wrinkles and facial hollows. In this procedure, fat is removed with a syringe from a patient's belly, buttocks, thigh, or hip. It is then cleaned of blood and other fluids and deposited in laugh lines, sunken chins, and hollow cheeks. The dermatologist kneads the fat evenly into wrinkles and furrows, which requires a great deal of skill and experience. Excess fat is stored and frozen, since the procedure has to be repeated on a monthly basis for about a year to be effective.

An advantage of fat injections over collagen injections is that the risk of allergic reaction is eliminated: Since your own fat is used, your body won't reject it. A disadvantage is that fat cells are not as controllable as collagen, which the dermatologist can more easily manipulate when she injects it. In addition, fat injections can be more painful than collagen injections, since a larger needle is required to accommodate the larger size of fat globules.

COSMETIC SURGERY

Every day thousands of women choose cosmetic surgery to smooth out wrinkles, remove fat deposits, and tighten sagging skin. As nearly 600,000 cosmetic operations are performed each year, creating a $250-million business, cosmetic surgery has become increasingly safer and more reliable. When chosen with discretion and performed properly, cosmetic surgery is an appropriate alternative. Yet cosmetic surgery—like any type of surgery—involves serious risks as well as benefits.

If you believe that cosmetic surgery will add to your self-esteem and vitality and ease your aging process, discuss the matter with your dermatologist or plastic surgeon: Cosmetic surgery may or may not be right for you. Examine your motives. Try not to be seduced, as are some women, into an ever escalating series of cosmetic operations and procedures, in an effort to mold yourself into society's arbitrary definition of ideal beauty.

A New Trend: Face-Lifts Before Fifty

It used to be mainly women in their fifties and sixties who sought out face-lifts. Today, almost a third of women opting for face-lifts are between the ages of thirty-five and fifty, according to the American Academy of Facial, Plastic and Reconstructive Surgery.

Some controversy exists about this new trend. Proponents say that face-lifts on younger women are not so drastic; women look subtly improved in appearance, but not drastically different. This type of rejuvenative surgery also should last longer when performed on younger women, when skin is more elastic. Older women, once they step on the face-lift treadmill, are in for frequent repeat appearances.

Others believe that a thirtysomething woman thinking about surgical rejuvenation should take a good look in the mirror. Relatively minor changes in your appearance at this age are not going to change your life. If you're using a face-lift as a means to solve problems with your career or relationships, or, worse yet, if you've fallen prey to our culture's obsession with the perfect image of Woman, then it's time to reconsider.

Yet many young women do make a valid case for rejuvenative surgery. For instance, if hormonal problems have triggered premature aging or if you have a congenital problem, the procedure's risks—which include bruising, scarring and rare instances of nerve damage—may be justified by the results.

Liposuction

Liposuction may well be one of the best remedies to get rid of sagging jowls or fat deposits under the chin. In this procedure, tiny incisions are made under the chin, and fat is suctioned out. The best candidate for this procedure is a woman in her thirties or forties whose skin still preserves a good degree of elasticity. Older women, who have little or no resilience left in the skin, must have excess skin removed with liposuction. Since this procedure, like any other, carries a certain amount of risk (such as infection), it should only be performed by a trained and experienced dermatologist or plastic surgeon.

HOW TO CHOOSE A DERMATOLOGIST

Many women who have a skin problem simply turn to the cosmetics counter or make a trip to the facial salon. This is fine for day-to-day skin care, but it can sometimes prove to be a very serious mistake. The FDA, after cracking down on the cosmetics industry in 1987, has adopted a more hands-off approach in recent years. Consequently, laws in some states permit potentially dangerous procedures, such as chemical peels, to be performed in salons and spas, even by persons who possess no medical degree or license.

If you're interested in exploring antiaging products beyond the realm of the purely cosmetic—whether alpha hydroxy acids, which many dermatologists believe can be overused or abused, or nonsurgical "face-lifts" such as chemical peels—it's crucially important to find a dermatologist or plastic surgeon who is both qualified and experienced.

For information on skin products and procedures, and for referrals to qualified doctors in your area, contact the American Academy of Dermatology or the American Academy of Facial,

Plastic and Reconstructive Surgery (see Appendix I: Resources, for addresses).

PROTECTING YOUR SKIN

In this chapter we've discussed the many ways in which you can care for your skin as you age. By now you know that much of the aging process is as avoidable as staying out of the sun or guarding your skin from the harmful ultraviolet rays of the sun. In the next chapter we will continue to explore the profoundly negative impact the sun can have on your skin and on your overall health. Exposure to sunlight does not only lead to premature aging; it can also lead to skin cancer.

CHAPTER 4

Skin cancer is "an undeclared epidemic," according to the American Academy of Dermatology. Skin cancers, or malignant skin growths, are the most widespread of all cancers, accounting for about a third of all reported malignancies in the United States today. In fact, skin cancer cases each year may be as common as all other cancers combined. At the current rate, one in every six Americans can expect to experience skin cancer at some point in his or her life. In 1994 doctors expect to diagnose 700,000 cases of nonmelanoma skin cancer, and some 32,000 cases of malignant melanoma. Nearly 7,000 melanoma deaths are expected.

SKIN CANCER IS PREVENTABLE

The good news is that almost all skin cancers are preventable. While most skin cancers appear in later life, the majority of your overall exposure to the sun usually takes place before age twenty. But whatever your age, both cumulative and intermittent exposure to the sun today increase your risk of developing skin cancer tomorrow, and are also the major causes of premature aging, wrinkling, and lining of your skin. The three best ways to protect yourself from the harmful rays of the sun are:

- Avoid peak hours of solar radiation.
- Use a broad spectrum sunscreen.
- Wear protective clothing.

THE THREE MAJOR TYPES OF SKIN CANCER

Skin cell growth begins in the epidermis, where healthy cells normally grow, divide, and replace themselves. This keeps the skin in good condition. Sometimes, however, skin cell growth becomes uncontrolled, leading to abnormal masses of tissue known as tumors.

Tumors can be either *benign* (noncancerous) or *malignant* (cancerous). Cancer cells in malignant tumors can break away from the original tumor and *metastasize,* or spread, through the blood and lymph systems, where they can form secondary, or metastatic, tumors.

There are three basic forms of skin cancer, and all are linked to cumulative exposure or overexposure to the sun. Basal cell and squamous cell carcinomas are referred to as nonmelanoma skin cancers to differentiate them from melanoma, which is the third and by far the most deadly variety of skin cancer.

SKIN CANCER AND THE SUN

The risk of developing nonmelanoma skin cancer is directly related to two major contributing factors:
- How many tans you get over the course of your lifetime
- How fair-skinned you are

Melanoma, on the other hand, appears to be linked to intermittent sunburns. People who have one or two severe sunburns in childhood may actually double their risk of developing melanoma in later life.

At highest risk for all types of skin cancer are fair-skinned individuals who burn or freckle easily in the sun (these people also often have blond or red hair and blue eyes). While no person or group is immune to skin cancer, blacks have the lowest incidence of all skin cancers because the high concentration of melanin in their skin protects them from ultraviolet radiation. It should also be kept in mind, however, that there are many shades of black skin, and a light-skinned black woman requires the same level of sun protection as a white woman with an olive skin tone.

The three basic sun-related types of skin cancer are:
- Basal cell carcinoma
- Squamous cell carcinoma
- Malignant melanoma

BASAL CELL CARCINOMA

Basal cell carcinoma accounts for about 90 percent of all skin cancers in the United States. Originating in the basal cells of the epidermis, this form of skin cancer first appears as small, fleshy nodules or bumps on frequently sun-exposed areas of your body, such as your hands, head, or neck. When these nodules appear on the trunk of the body, as they occasionally do, the growths are flat.

Fortunately, basal cell tumors are slow-growing and rarely metastasize, or spread to other parts of the body. It may take months or even years for a basal cell carcinoma to reach a diameter of a half inch. Like most skin cancers, basal cell carcinomas most commonly affect fair-skinned people who do not tan easily; significant amounts of melanin in dark-skinned women offers greater protection from ultraviolet light, which makes these women less likely to develop tumors.

Diagnosis and Treatment

Basal cell carcinoma has a cure rate of 95 percent when diagnosed and treated at an early stage, according to the American Academy of Dermatology. Yet if not treated properly, these tumors may begin to bleed and crust over again and again. As slowly as they do spread, it is eventually possible that a neglected basal cell carcinoma may extend below the skin and cause damage to the underlying bone.

Dermatologists can often identify a nonmelanoma skin cancer on sight, and a biopsy is usually done in your doctor's office, under local anesthesia, to remove all or part of the growth. Often a nonmelanoma skin cancer can be completely removed at the time of the biopsy, and no further treatment is necessary.

After the biopsy, a pathologist will study the cells under a microscope to determine whether the growth is benign or cancerous. *Curettage* is the procedure most often used to treat basal cell carcinoma, when a biopsy is not successful in removing all cancer cells. In this procedure, the area is numbed with a local anesthetic, and the cancer is scooped out with a sharp, spoon-shaped instrument called a curette. In a process known as *electrodesiccation,* an electric current may then be applied to the area to destroy any remaining cancer cells. This combination of curettage and electrodesiccation is known as *electrosurgery.*

SQUAMOUS CELL CARCINOMA

Squamous cell carcinoma, the second most common type of skin cancer, may first appear as a pink, tan, or brown bump or patch on a sun-exposed area of your skin. Actinic keratosis, a precancerous condition of gray, red, or brown scaly patches on the skin, often leads to squamous cell carcinoma.

Tumors that begin in the squamous cells of the epidermis grow more rapidly than those of basal cells and are commonly found on the face, lips, mouth, ears, and the back of the hands. In their early stages, squamous cell tumors may be difficult to detect. At first they are firm to the touch; but eventually they form a central crust, which becomes ulcerated and causes inflammation of surrounding skin.

While also relatively slow to spread—especially in comparison with the aggressive growth rate of deadly melanoma—squamous cell carcinomas are more red and swollen and tend to grow faster than basal cell carcinomas. Like basal cell carcinomas, squamous cell carcinomas most commonly affect fair-skinned people who do not tan easily, and are rarely a problem for dark-skinned women.

Diagnosis and Treatment

The cure rate for squamous cell carcinoma, like that of basal cell carcinoma, is an encouraging 95 percent or better when the cancer is found and treated at an early stage. Overall, only 2 percent of squamous cell carcinomas spread to other organs. But of special medical concern are squamous cell carcinomas that develop on the lips or in burn or X-ray scars; up to 20 percent of these tumors metastasize and invade underlying tissues.

Dermatologists can usually identify squamous cell carcinomas on sight, just as they can basal cell carcinomas. A biopsy performed under local anesthesia in the doctor's office can often remove the entire growth. Following the biopsy, a pathologist will study the cells under a microscope to determine whether the growth is benign or cancerous, and whether additional treatment is needed to remove the entire cancer.

Further Treatments for Nonmelanoma Skin Cancers

At times, additional treatment is required for nonmelanoma skin cancers. These include:

- **Cryosurgery** Also known as cryotherapy, a technique in which liquid nitrogen is sprayed on the growth to freeze and kill abnormal cells. Used to treat precancerous actinic keratoses, small and well-defined basal cell carcinomas, and some squamous cell carcinomas.
- **Mohs' technique** A highly specialized type of surgery in which a cancer is removed one thin layer at a

time. Especially effective in curing hard-to-treat or recurrent nonmelanoma skin cancers.

- **Radiation therapy** A method in which high-energy
rays are used to kill cancer cells. Often used to treat
nonmelanoma skin cancers that occur on the head or
neck.
- **Topical chemotherapy** The application of the anticancer drug 5-fluorouracil (5-U) as a cream or solution on a daily basis to a growth for several weeks.
Used to treat actinic keratoses and some superficial
basal cell and squamous cell carcinomas.

MELANOMA

Melanoma, which is also known as malignant or cutaneous
melanoma, is the deadliest and most virulent form of skin cancer. Overall, the five-year survival rate for skin melanoma is
84.1 percent. But if the cancer has spread to distant lymph
nodes, tissues, or organs, the five-year rate of survival drops to a
frightening 14.2 percent.

While relatively rare in comparison with nonmelanoma skin
cancers, the number of people who develop this life-threatening
skin cancer each year is increasing at an alarming rate of 7 percent each year—far faster than any other type of cancer. According to a 1994 Connecticut State Health Department study, from
1989 to 1991, eight Connecticut coastal communities with public beaches had 64 percent more cases of malignant cancer than
would be expected. Incidence rates of melanoma have been increasing steadily among women aged twenty to forty-four. And
today one in every hundred Americans can expect to contract
melanoma at some point in his or her life. Melanoma is most
common in fair-skinned people who live in geographical locations where the sunlight is most intense. Yet unlike nonmelanoma skin cancer, melanoma occurs less rarely in people
with dark brown or black skin, usually under the nails, in the
mouth, on the palms of hands, or the soles of feet.

Melanoma, Dysplastic Nevi, and the Sun

Malignant melanoma is an aggressive cancer that originates in the melanocytes, the cells in the epidermis that contain and produce melanin (the pigment that gives skin its color). A mole or brown spot—in dermatological terms, a *nevus*—occurs when pigment-rich melanocytes form a cluster. When a mole changes color or shape, you are at serious risk for skin melanoma and should see your doctor immediately. The colors can range from brown and black to red and white, and the moles are not necessarily located in areas exposed to the sun.

Approximately one in every ten people has unusual moles, which dermatologists refer to as *dysplastic nevi*. Dysplastic nevi are more likely than normal moles to develop into malignant melanomas. Although not everyone who has dysplastic nevi develops melanoma, it's important that all abnormal moles be closely monitored by both your dermatologist and yourself through regular examinations.

In contrast to nonmelanoma skin cancers, which are caused by cumulative exposure to the sun over one's lifetime, melanomas appear to be linked to intermittent sunburns. The dysplastic nevi that develop into melanomas usually grow on parts of the body not frequently exposed to direct sunlight: the back, the trunk, arms, and legs. One theory explaining why this occurs is that these areas suffer the most severe burns when exposed. Research shows that experiencing even one or two sunburns as a child or teenager may double your chance of developing of melanoma in later life. (See Figure 2, pp. 52–53.)

Are You at Risk for Melanoma?

Certain people are at a greater risk for developing melanoma. If you are one of them, it's especially important to be familiar with the warning signs of melanoma, to visit your dermatologist on a regular basis, and to conduct monthly skin self-exams. Learning about the prevention and early detection of skin cancer is important for everyone, but particularly for those who have one or more of these risk factors:

- Dysplastic nevi, or unusual moles
- A large number of moles (the normal range is considered to be between 10 and 40)
- A personal history of skin cancer
- A close relative who has had skin cancer (about 10 percent of melanomas run in families)
- A history of one or more severe, blistering sunburns as a child or teenager
- Fair skin that burns or freckles easily
- If you live in an area with a high level of UV radiation (for example, in the southern United States)

COMMON BENIGN SKIN GROWTHS: THE BARNACLES OF AGING

Not all skin growths are cancerous. Many are harmless, and most occur as we age. Genetic predisposition, exposure to the sun, and hormonal changes may all play a role in the development of these barnacles of aging. While moles are often harmless, we do not list them here since they have the potential of developing into skin cancer and should therefore be closely monitored by both you and your dermatologist.

Common benign skin growths include:

- **Cysts** Cysts are small closed sacs within hair follicles that contain keratin, cellular debris, and oil gland secretions. Cysts can become inflamed, infected and uncomfortable, and may result in lasting scars. *Milia,* which resemble whiteheads, and *open follicular cysts,* which look like blackheads, are two common forms

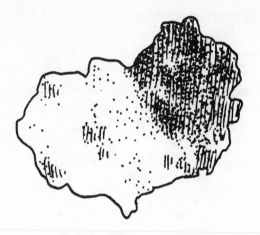

1. Uneven shape

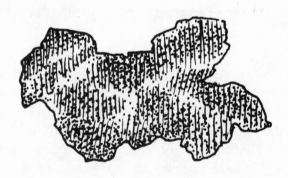

2. Irregular borders

FIGURE 2A-D Danger Signs in Moles

Abnormal or unusual moles, called atypical nevi or dysplastic nevi, are prone to develop melanoma. Consult your dermatologist if you detect moles on your body that display any of the above abnormal traits.

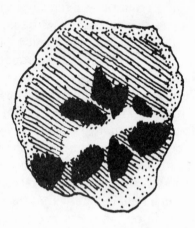

3. A mixture of pigments

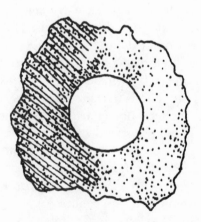

4. Larger than 6 mm (bigger
than the top of a pencil
eraser)

of cyst. Your dermatologist can surgically remove or drain most cysts under local anesthesia.

- **Flat Warts** Flat warts, or verruca plana, are so-named for their smooth, flat appearance. Warts are a very common skin tumor, caused by a viral infection, the papilloma virus, and different types of warts appear on different parts of the body. Flat warts on the face and neck are usually smooth, velvety, and regularly shaped. These warts are also commonly found on the backs of hands and legs. While it is often desirable to remove warts for cosmetic reasons, it's important to keep in mind that warts are an essentially harmless condition, and any measures that you and your dermatologist decide on to remove them should be equally benign. Flat warts are sometimes confused with seborrheic dermatoses.

- **Lipomas** Lipomas are fatty deposits that may resemble sebaceous cysts. Lipomas are generally harmless skin tumors that cause no symptoms. If they cause pain or cosmetic embarrassment, lipomas can be removed by your dermatologist through a small incision under local anesthesia.

- **Seborrheic Keratoses** Seborrheic keratoses are layered and greasy brown, yellow, or gray scaly patches on the skin. These harmless growths range in size from the diameter of a quarter to many inches across. Because they are located on the surface of the skin, seborrheic keratoses can be easily removed by your dermatologist through curettage or chemical applications under local anesthesia. Seborrheic keratoses rarely develop into skin cancer.

- **Skin Tags** Skin tags, or papillomas, are fine stalks of skin that may be flesh-colored or slightly pigmented. These are harmless growths that commonly occur during pregnancy and in diabetic or postmenopausal women. Skin tags are most common on the neck, but may develop on the chest, under the breasts, on the inner thighs, or on the face. Small skin tags can be removed by your dermatologist with special scissors, while broad or twisted skin tags may require electrosurgery or cryosurgery.

- **Solar Lentigines** These harmless flat, brown marks, which are also known as age or liver spots, commonly appear on the face, hands, back, and feet of middle-aged and older individuals. They are caused by cumulative exposure to the sun over the course of one's lifetime. If you find them cosmetically unappealing, an over-the-counter concealer may be helpful. Alternatively, your dermatologist may prescribe Retin-A or use techniques such as cryosurgery or electrosurgery to remove solar lentigines.

Whole Body Exams

In an important new trend in dermatology, doctors periodically inspect your whole body for any changes, such as a new mole or blemish or variations in the surface of a mole. A common site for melanomas is on the back, for example, where the disease can progress unnoticed for long periods. Fortunately, skin cancers can be easily detected in whole body exams, and your best defense lies in early detection and removal of a tumor. Even malignant melanoma can be treated successfully when caught in its early stages.

The Benefits of Skin Self-Examination

Dermatologists also recommend that you perform your own periodic skin self-examinations. Although the benefits of self-examination are widely recognized in the detection of health problems such as breast cancer, the American Academy of Dermatology is campaigning for more attention to be paid to the importance of self-exams in the detection of melanoma.

A ten-minute self-examination each month is one major way you can participate in the crucial early detection of melanoma. If you have a higher than average risk for melanoma, it's important to be especially vigilant—but regular skin self-exams are a good idea for everyone.

Remember that melanoma usually begins on the surface of the skin. Closely monitor any new spot on your skin or any change in an existing mole. Skin lesions that fail to heal and bleeding or festering moles should be examined at once by your dermatologist.

The best time to do a skin self-exam is after a bath or shower. Good lighting is a must. Learn where your moles, blemishes, and "beauty marks" are located, and how they normally look and feel. Any changes call for an immediate appointment with your dermatologist.Here's how to perform a monthly self-examination of your skin:

1. Check yourself from head to toe. Examine the front and back of your body in a full-length mirror. Then raise your arms and look at your right and left sides.
2. Bend your elbows, and take a careful look at your upper arms, forearms, palms, and fingernails.
3. Check the front, back, and sides of your legs. Look at the spaces between your toes and soles.
4. Examine the back of your neck and your scalp with a hand mirror. Part hair for a closer look.
5. Check your back and buttocks with a hand mirror.

(See Figure 3, p. 58–59.)

Diagnosis and Treatment

An average of 85 percent of people with melanoma are diagnosed at an early stage when the tumor is thin and cancer cells have not yet grown downward from the skin's surface. Melanoma is almost always curable at this early stage, via surgical removal. Chemotherapy and radiation, while useful treatments for nonmelanoma skin cancers, have little or no impact on deadly melanoma. Experimental melanoma vaccines may help a small percentage of melanoma patients, and researchers are making progress in linking a defective gene to melanoma. In the meantime, however, early detection and removal continue to be by far the most effective defenses against malignant melanoma.

The early detection of melanoma is critical, since once this virulent cancer appears it can spread quickly though the lymphatic system and bloodstream to other parts of the body. In fact, malignant melanoma metastasizes faster than any other form of cancer. Many people whose melanoma is diagnosed after it has already spread will die within a year.

If your doctor suspects that an abnormal mole is an indication of melanoma, you will need to have a biopsy (which is usually performed in your doctor's office under local anesthesia) to remove all or part of the mole. Later, a skin pathologist will examine the tissue under a microscope to determine if cancer cells are present.

OTHER TYPES OF SKIN CANCER

Less common types of skin cancer are *Kaposi's sarcoma* and *mycosis fungoides*. You don't have to have AIDS to have these tumors. These are cancers that have been around for centuries, but they are much more common in the HIV-positive population today.

Kaposi's sarcoma is a type of cancer that develops on the skin of people who have a weakened immune system, especially due to AIDS (Acquired Immune Deficiency Syndrome). Mycosis

Here's how to perform a monthly self-examination of your skin.

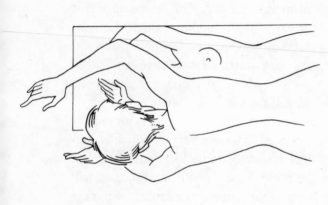

1) Check yourself from head to toe. Examine the front and back of your body in a full-length mirror. Then raise your arms and look at your right and left sides.

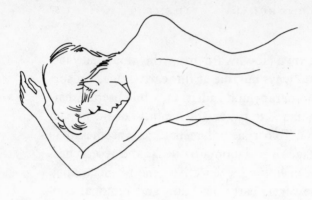

2) Bend your elbows and take a careful look at your upper arms, forearms, palms, and fingernails.

FIGURE 3A-E Performing a Skin Self-Exam

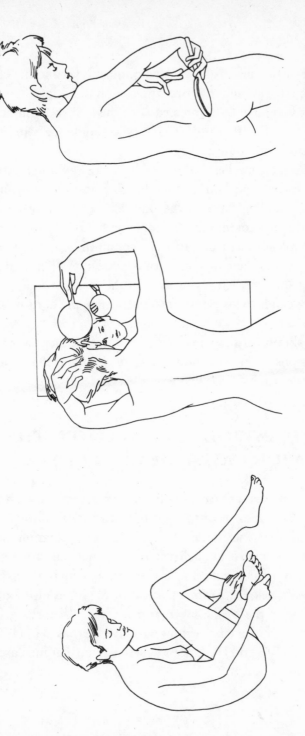

3) Check the front, back, and sides of your legs. Look at the spaces between your toes and soles.

4) Examine the back of your neck and your scalp with a hand mirror. Part hair for a closer look.

5) Check your back and buttocks with a hand mirror.

fungoides, also known as T-cell lymphoma, is yet another cancer of the immune system that first appears on the skin. (If you suspect that you have been infected with the human immunodeficiency virus [HIV] that causes AIDS, you should see your doctor immediately to initiate an aggressive course of treatment.)

As the name implies, HIV severely impairs your immune system and leaves your body vulnerable to a host of opportunistic diseases, including those of the skin. Skin cancers, rashes, and growths appear commonly in people with AIDS who are often resistant to treatment due to their compromised immune systems. At present there is no cure for AIDS, but millions of dollars are being spent on AIDS research. In the meantime, aggressive treatment can help keep HIV infection and many of its manifestations in check.

Any skin metastases may also be a sign of internal cancer. These lesions are most common on the scalp, but may also appear on the trunk or elsewhere on the body.

ULTRAVIOLET RADIATION: THE MAJOR CAUSE OF SKIN CANCER

Each time you are exposed to the sunlight you are also exposed to two types of ultraviolet (UV) radiation: ultraviolet B (UVB) and ultraviolet A (UVA). Both types of radiation, invisible to the human eye, are believed to play important roles in the development of skin cancer and premature aging of the skin.

A third type of radiation given off by the sun is ultraviolet C (UVC). So far the ozone layer protects us by absorbing UVC rays, but as the ozone layer thins we may be exposed to UVC, in addition to UVB and UVA rays, which may further increase our risk of skin cancer.

UVB RADIATION DAMAGE

UVB rays are short, energetic wavelengths that have long been associated with sunburn and skin damage. Exposure to UVB rays is a major risk factor for skin cancer, especially basal and squamous cell carcinomas. This type of radiation is most intense between the hours of 10 A.M. and 3 P.M. standard time, in the summer months, and in climates closest to the equator. In the United States, for example, skin cancer is more common in southern states such as Florida and Texas than it is in Maine or Minnesota, where the sun's rays are not as strong.

Short UVB rays penetrate the top layer of skin, damaging DNA, thickening the epidermis, and stimulating the production of melanin (the pigment your body produces in an attempt to protect itself from radiation). In other words, by the time your skin begins to pinken, tan, or burn, it is already experiencing damage from the sun. Remember: There is no such thing as a healthy tan.

UVA RADIATION DAMAGE

For many years experts focused attention on UVB as the major risk factor in skin damage. Over the last ten years, however, suspicion has developed that UVA rays are not the safe tanning rays we thought they were. There is concern that UVA radiation may be, in its own way, just as dangerous as UVB.

Today scientists are considering the role of UVA rays in causing the most virulent form of skin cancer: melanoma. UVA's elongated rays take longer than those of UVB to produce a burn, but they also penetrate more deeply into the lower layer of your skin. UVA is thought to damage collagen and elastin, the substances that keep skin young and firm. Both UVB and UVA rays suppress your skin's immune function and, together, may contribute to melanoma growth.

UVA rays are also more abundant and more persistent than

UVB rays. Many of the shorter UVB rays are absorbed by the ozone layer and do not reach the earth's surface, but longer UVA rays are not absorbed as they pass through the atmosphere. They are more constant in intensity, penetrating all areas of the earth, all day long, all year long. The greater wavelength of UVA even allows them to penetrate glass (UVB rays cannot do this).

ULTRAVIOLET DAMAGE IS CUMULATIVE

Although most skin cancers appear in later years, the sun's damaging effects begin at an early age. In fact, as much as 80 percent of lifetime exposure to the sun and resulting damage takes place before the age of twenty. In addition to increasing risk of skin cancer, long-term exposure to UVB and UVA rays leads to premature aging of your skin, which means wrinkling, sagging, and the development of age or liver spots. It is also thought to contribute to cataracts and other eye problems as we age, according to the American Optometric Association.

AGE SPOTS AND THE SUN

Whatever name they go by, age or liver spots are not caused by either the natural aging process or by liver problems. *Solar lentigines* is the dermatological term for these harmless marks, which are actually a direct result of your cumulative exposure to the sun over the years.

If you exercise good sun protection, you can avoid developing age spots. If you do develop them and find them to be a cosmetic nuisance, you can use a concealer. You might also ask your dermatologist if Retin-A is an appropriate treatment for you. Applying Retin-A over a period of months can make age spots fade or even disappear.

THE SUN'S RAYS CAN BE DECEPTIVE

Many people mistakenly believe that they cannot get a sunburn on an overcast day. However, although it is easier to burn on a hot day when the sunlight intensifies the effects of UV radiation, up to 80 percent of UV rays are capable of penetrating clouds. Your best bet on a cloudy day is to continue to take normal precautions, such as limiting your exposure to the sun during peak hours and using a broad spectrum sunscreen.

Lightweight summer clothing is often thought to boost sun protection. Yet true protection is offered only by tightly woven protective clothing that is specially designed to block the harmful rays of the sun. Many hats and visors leave the lower half of your face—as well as your sensitive ears—exposed to possible sun damage. Likewise, the sun's rays are fully capable of penetrating a white T-shirt, which provides an average SPF of only 8. If the T-shirt is wet from perspiration or swimming, that SPF is reduced to about 5. (Read more about SPFs, or Sun Protection Factors, later in this chapter.)

Even sitting in the shade is no guarantee of protection against tanning or sunburn. Beach umbrellas, for example, are sometimes thought to counter the harmful effects of the sun. But while they may offer a degree of protection, UV rays can still bounce off sand and water to burn the person lounging comfortably underneath.

Hikers and skiers should take extra care to protect themselves from the harmful effects of the sun. At high altitudes there is less atmosphere to block the ultraviolet rays of the sun. Wind can worsen the effects of the sun, while shiny snow can reflect up to 80 percent of the sun's rays.

WHO IS AFFECTED BY THE SUN?

With the decreased ozone layer, everyone is more at risk of the harmful effects of the sun. Skin damage from UV radiation varies widely according to skin type and color. Fair-skinned people are most vulnerable to skin damage, although UVA rays can penetrate even dark skin protected with melanin. Your location, the time of day, the season, and the amount of sun exposure you have received recently also play a role in determining your present susceptibility to the sun.

The American Academy of Dermatology has classified five skin types, which are ranked according to susceptibility to burning when exposed to the sun:

- **Type I** Extremely sensitive. A fair skin that never tans and burns immediately. If you have fair skin, blue or green eyes, red or blond hair, and freckles, you are at the highest risk of damage from exposure to the sun.
- **Type II** Very sensitive. A fair skin that burns easily and tans minimally.
- **Type III** Sensitive. A somewhat fair skin that burns moderately and tans gradually to a light brown. Individuals usually have light-brown hair and blue, green or brown eyes.
- **Type IV** Minimally sensitive. This is a skin type that tans well to a dark brown and burns only occasionally. If you have olive skin, brown hair, and brown eyes, you probably have this type of skin.
- **Type V** Not sensitive. Individuals with very dark skin, hair, and eyes almost never burn.

LIGHT SENSITIVITY AND
MEDICATION

Be especially careful about your exposure to the sun when you are taking medication. The combination of some medications and sunlight can increase your sensitivity to the sun, increasing your risk of adverse reactions ranging from rashes, sunburns, and premature aging to cataracts, damaged immunity, and skin cancer.

Medications that can cause these types of photosensitivity include:

- Antihistamines
- Dandruff shampoos
- Nonsteroidal anti-inflammatory drugs (or NSAIDs, such as ibuprofen)
- Oral contraceptives
- Psoralens
- Sulfa drugs
- Tetracycline
- Thiazide diuretics
- Tranquilizers
- Tricyclic antidepressants

HOW TO PREVENT SKIN CANCER

Protecting your skin from the sun is the most effective way to prevent skin damage—damage that can eventually result in skin cancer and the wrinkled, leathery skin of premature aging. But this *doesn't* mean that you have to spend the rest of your life indoors. You don't have to give up your favorite outdoor pastimes, whether they be tennis, golf, or swimming. Whenever you go outside, and whatever you do, simply exercise sensible precautions to protect yourself from the harmful rays of the sun and keep your skin healthy.

The three main precautions you should take are:

- Avoid midday sun.
- Wear protective clothing and hat.
- Use a broad spectrum sunscreen or sunblock.

AVOID MIDDAY SUN

The bottom line is that it's best to limit the time you spend in the sun between the hours of 10 A.M. and 3 P.M. standard time, when the sun's UVB rays are strongest. Try to go for your run or schedule your tennis game in the early morning or late afternoon. Keep in mind that the sun's rays are most powerful in the summer, when the heat of the sun intensifies the impact of UV radiation. In terms of location, the closer you are to the equator, the stronger the rays of the sun. Whatever time of year, UVA rays are strong all day. So other forms of protection are important as well.

WEAR PROTECTIVE CLOTHING

Wear a broad-brimmed hat, a long-sleeved shirt, long pants, and sunglasses when you go out in the sun. Many garments allow ultraviolet light to penetrate. If you have fair skin, or are going outside at midday, it is especially important to apply sunscreen *under* sheer clothing.

Some companies—such as Sun Precautions in Seattle, Washington—offer cool and lightweight clothing that has the ability to block over 97 percent of the sun's harmful ultraviolet rays. The more tightly woven the hat or cover-up, the greater the protection.

USE A BROAD SPECTRUM SUNSCREEN OR SUNBLOCK

The American Academy of Dermatology recommends that we all use a broad spectrum sunscreen or sunblock with the correct Sun Protection Factor (SPF) for our particular skin type. "Broad spectrum" indicates protection from UVA as well as UVB rays. An SPF of 15 or higher is also advised, and those with sensitive skin should be certain to use a PABA-free product. The sunscreen or sunblock should be evenly applied at least fifteen minutes before exposure to the sun to allow time for protective ingredients to interact with the skin.

Sunscreen or Sunblock?

In the not so distant past, conventional sunscreens offered protection against only UVB rays, while sunblock (that bright white zinc oxide on the lifeguard's nose, for example) reflected away *all* harmful UV rays of the sun. Yet as experts have come to realize the importance of protecting your skin from UVA as well as UVB rays, the distinction between sunscreens and sunblocks has blurred.

Today it is not so important that you choose sunscreen or sunblock; the key is to use a "broad-based" or "broad spectrum" sun protection product, one that guards you against the harmful effects of both UVB and UVA radiation. Many manufacturers are in the process of developing sunblocks that are less conspicuous than that old-fashioned white ointment by blending them with creamier bases. Other manufacturers are adding additional protective chemicals to sunscreens to provide UVA as well as UVB protection.

Common Ingredients in Sun Preparations

The most effective sunscreens and sunblocks list one of these three ingredients on the label: benzophene (which protects skin from UVB and UVA rays); avobenzene (which deflects UVA rays); or titanium dioxide (which blocks everything). If you have especially sensitive skin, you may be allergic to some of the chemicals in conventional sunscreens, such as PABA or oxybenzone. To prevent a sensitivity reaction, do a patch test before using a new sunscreen. Apply to the inside of the wrist a day before you want to use it more widely. If a rash develops, switch to a different sun care product (for example, one that is PABA-free).

Translating Sun Protection Jargon

It's important to read labels carefully to get the broad spectrum protection you need and the appropriate SPF for your skin type. But as the nature of sun protection has grown more complex, so has the language that describes it. Here are a few definitions that may help you sort out what's right for you:

- **Sunscreen**   A cream or lotion containing invisible ingredients that protect your skin by absorbing the harmful ultraviolet rays of the sun. Formerly, sunscreens offered protection only against UVB rays; today's broad spectrum sunscreens extend protection to include UVA rays.

- **Sunblock**   A substance that protects your skin from the harmful rays of the sun by reflecting UVB and UVA rays. Sunblocks contain active ingredients such as titanium dioxide and zinc oxide—often white, opaque substances that are not absorbed by the skin. Today's formulas have been redesigned to contain absorbers that make sunblock appear less visible and thus more attractive to use.

- **Broad spectrum sunscreen or sunblock**   Conventional sunscreens are effective only against UVB rays; broad-based or broad spectrum sunscreens and sunblocks offer protection against both UVB and UVA rays.

- **Waterproof sunscreen or sunblock** Waterproof sun preparations are effective in the water for approximately 80 minutes. If you towel dry, you must reapply for full protection.
- **Sun Protection Factor (SPF)** A scale that rates the level of protection sunscreens provide from the UVB rays of the sun. The SPF provides a measurement of how long you can spend in the sun without burning. For example, if you are a fair-skinned person, you might ordinarily turn pink in about 10 minutes. This pink tinge is actually the beginning of skin damage. But if you use a sunscreen with an SPF of 15, your skin is protected for 150 minutes before skin damage occurs.

  The American Academy of Dermatology recommends daily use of a broad spectrum sunscreen with an SPF of 15 or higher.
- **PABA-free** Many common sun preparations contain PABA, or para-aminobenzoic acid. Since PABA often causes allergic reactions, those with sensitive skin should choose PABA-free products.
- **Suntan lotion** Designed to moisturize the skin and permit tanning, it offers little or no sun protection and is not recommended.

AN INDEX FOR SAFETY IN THE SUN

In June 1994, in an effort to help people avoid skin cancer, the National Weather Service began issuing a new daily solar warning index, devised by the Environmental Protection Agency and the National Oceanic and Atmospheric Administration. These daily forecasts of ultraviolet exposure cover at least one city in every state and determine the amount of dangerous ultraviolet light from the sun that will hit the earth's surface around noon of the following day.

The risk categories are:

- **0–2:** Minimal risk. While very fair-skinned people may burn in 30 minutes, those less susceptible to skin damage may be safe for up to two hours at this level of solar exposure.
- **3–4:** Low risk. Fair-skinned individuals are safe for some 15 to 20 minutes in the sun, whereas those with more protective skin types are apt to experience sun damage in 75 to 90 minutes.
- **5–6:** Moderate risk. Fair-skinned people are safe for only 10 to 12 minutes. Those with darker skin may be protected for up to 50 to 60 minutes.
- **7–9:** High risk. If you are fair-skinned, you are safe for only 7 to 8½ minutes at this level of intensity. Those less susceptible to burning may last for 33 to 40 minutes.
- **10 and above:** Very high risk. If you are fair-skinned and need to go outside when the sun is at this level, you should remain exposed for only 4 to 6 minutes. Those with the most protection may remain in the sun for 20 to 30 minutes.

SOOTHING A SUNBURN

If, despite all the precautions you take, you end up with a sunburn, try these soothing tips:

- Apply cool compresses to burned areas.
- Take a cool bath.
- Drink lots of liquids to replace depleted body fluids.
- Never apply greasy ointments or butter, which seal in heat and make sunburn more painful.

- Apply aloe vera or over-the-counter sunburn spray to relieve inflammation, promote healing, and take the sting out of the burn.
- Take two aspirin (children and teenagers should take acetaminophen instead, because of the link between aspirin and the rare but life-threatening disease Reyes Syndrome).
- In the case of a severe sunburn accompanied by fever and blistered skin, see your doctor for medical treatment. Sunburns in infants are and should be treated as medical emergencies.

IS AN ARTIFICIAL TAN SAFE?

The answer to this question is: It depends on how you get it. Artificial sources of UV radiation can be just as deadly as the sun. Self-tanning cosmetics, on the other hand, are a safe way to give your skin the "healthy" glow you crave, without exposing yourself to dangerous UV radiation. Over-the-counter melanin promoters can activate the production of your own melanin cells.

The major users of artificial tanning devices such as tanning booths and beds, reflectors, and sunlamps, are teenagers and young women. Like natural sunlight, artificial tanning devices emit ultraviolet rays. Ultraviolet rays, whether they are UVA or UVB and whether they are from natural or artificial sources, cause skin damage that can lead to skin cancer. Despite its apparent cosmetic appeal to many people, this type of tan is a sign that damage to the skin has occurred and may cause serious health problems down the line.

Because people everywhere are coming to realize that our days of carefree sunbathing are over, cosmetic companies are jumping into the fray with a wide variety of self-tanning products. Self-action tanning lotions, creams, and sprays are flooding the marketplace, promising relatively danger-free tans in shades ranging from medium to dark. Many self-tanners are fine-tuned to match their color to your skin tone, and contain sunscreen and moisturizers.

A SPECIAL GUIDE TO SUN PROTECTION FOR CHILDREN

The best time to begin preventing skin cancer is in childhood. Children should be taught good sun protection habits just as they are taught the follies of smoking and the benefits of wearing seatbelts and bicycle helmets.

Children spend three times as much time in the sun as adults do, and experts estimate that 80 percent of a person's lifetime exposure to cancer-causing ultraviolet radiation takes place before the age of twenty. Sun exposure takes place whether your child is lying on the beach, playing sports, or mowing the lawn. So while outdoor activities are a big part of childhood, it is important to remember that all sun exposure can be damaging—no matter where or how it takes place.

Parents and caretakers of children should routinely apply a sunscreen with an SPF of at least 25 every time children go outdoors. Whenever possible, cover up your child with a broad-brimmed hat, a long-sleeved shirt, and long pants. Parents should advocate sun-protective school-yard coverage. Whenever possible, do not allow your child to play outside when the sun's rays are at their most intense, between 10 A.M. and 3 P.M.

As for very young children, keep them out of the sun! Sunscreens should not even be used until babies are at least six months old, since chemicals in them can irritate the delicate skin of newborns. The developing eyes of infants are also so sensitive that experts recommend that children of this age be kept out of the sun altogether. Shade is the best protection for babies. A sunburn, painful at any time, can be a serious medical emergency in the first year of life.

CHILDREN AT RISK IN THE SUN

It's never too early to begin protecting your children from the ultraviolet rays of the sun. Do not assume that because your child is dark-skinned, no precautions need be taken. Children of color can also get sunburned and can also get skin cancer—although not as often as light-skinned children. The most vulnerable children have:
- Blue, green, or gray eyes
- Fair skin or freckles
- A tendency to burn before tanning or never tan at all
- Birthmarks
- A tendency to develop dysplastic nevi
- Moles or skin blemishes that show abnormal changes
- A family history of skin cancer

HOW TO PROTECT YOUR SKIN FROM THE SUN

Following is a summary of the guidelines you should follow to protect your skin from intense ultraviolet radiation:
- Plan outdoor activities for early morning or late afternoon to minimize your exposure to the sun during midday.

- Wear a broad-brimmed hat, a long-sleeved shirt, and long pants.
- Walk on the shady side of the street.
- Use a broad spectrum sunscreen or sunblock with an SPF of at least 15 whenever you go outside. Fair-skinned individuals and children should use an SPF of 25 to 30.
- Apply a liberal amount of broad spectrum sunblock before each exposure to the sun. About one ounce spread evenly over your body constitutes an average application. Unfortunately, many people use considerably less and are not protecting themselves adequately.
- Reapply sunscreen at least every two hours. If you swim or perspire a great deal, apply sunscreen more often.
- Use waterproof sunscreen if you frequently go swimming or perspire a great deal.
- Don't forget to apply sun protection on cloudy days, or even when you're in the shade. Surfaces such as sand, water, snow, and concrete reflect the sun's rays.
- Remember to apply sunscreen when engaging in high-altitude activities such as hiking and skiing.
- If you experience a sensitive reaction to a sunscreen or sunblock, choose a different product.
- Avoid artificial sources of ultraviolet radiation, such as tanning booths, tanning beds, reflectors, and sunlamps.
- Ask your doctor or pharmacist about the possibility of increased photosensitivity due to the medications you take.
- Teach children sun protection at an early age.
- Keep newborns out of the sun.

MAINTAINING HEALTHY SKIN

In this chapter you have learned that it is possible to prevent most cases of skin cancer and that early detection and diagnosis can lead to successful treatment and cures. In the chapters that follow you will see that this same strategy applies to effectively coping with a wide variety of skin problems, from skin rashes to viral, bacterial, fungal, and parasitic infections.

CHAPTER 5

COPING WITH SKIN RASHES

Almost everyone experiences difficulty with his or her skin at some point in life, and rashes—often uncomfortable, at times noticeable, and occasionally disfiguring—can pose emotional as well as physical anguish. In this chapter we'll discuss noninfectious and noncontagious skin rashes, which range from mild and easily treated cases of acne to severe cases of psoriasis that may call for hospitalization. Dermatologists refer to these rashes as "inflammatory," since they are most often due to acute or chronic inflammation of the skin.

While rashes due to infections of the skin are clearly caused by a virus, fungus, bacterial, or parasitic infection, the causes of most noninfectious rashes continue to elude medical science. A wide variety of factors may contribute to these conditions, such as hormonal imbalances, follicle dysfunction, allergies, stress, and genetic influences. Here we'll discuss the causes, symptoms, and treatments of common noninfectious skin rashes.

ACNE

People who suffer from acne—a frustrating, embarrassing, and sometimes scarring skin disorder—constitute about 20 percent of all those who seek treatment for skin problems. Each year nearly 17 million Americans suffer from this inflammatory condition of the skin (which is medically known as *acne vulga-*

ris), and 4.5 million people visit dermatologists due to acne-
related problems.

Although acne is often thought to be a problem of adolescence, it is a condition that can affect people of all ages. Later in
life, acne outbreaks may be set off or aggravated by such factors
as stress, menstrual periods, steroids, or the use of oral contraceptives. Fortunately, there are many actions you can take to
control acne that we'll discuss later. First, let's examine the
sources of acne.

WHAT CAUSES ACNE?

While the exact cause of acne vulgaris is unknown, it appears to be linked to hormonal factors. Acne occurs when a fatty
acid called *sebum* is overproduced by the sebaceous glands in
small openings in the skin known as *follicles* or *pores*. In addition, there is excess keratin scaling in these pores. Sebum normally supplies moisture to your skin, helping to keep it smooth
and wrinkle-free. But when too much sebum is present, follicles
become clogged, and bacteria multiply in tiny blocked channels.
These channels soon become inflamed and swollen, and sometimes fill with pus.

While acne can and does occur at any age, it is most common
during adolescence when hormones seem to run amok. At the
onset of sexual maturity, both males and females secrete increased amounts of hormones called *androgens,* which in turn
overstimulate the sebaceous glands.

Severe acne is much more common in teenage boys than in
teenage girls, probably due to the fact that boys secrete more
androgens. But later in life, this trend reverses: Adult women
tend to develop acne more often than adult men, although not
nearly so often as teenagers of either sex. Experts speculate that
acne in adult women is due to an increase both in hormonal

activity during premenstrual flares and in the production of adrenal androgens as a result of chronic stress.

Race also seems to play a role in acne, which is more severe in whites than in the black population. The good news is that most cases of acne eventually clear up as hormonal activity evens out in your twenties, and as the aging process gives you sturdier skin that acts as a more effective barrier to acne.

While acne in adults is less severe than in teenagers, in both groups acne has been linked to problems with self-esteem, self-image, embarrassment, depression, anger, and frustration.

SKIN DISORDERS: THE EMOTIONAL TOLL ON YOUR LIFE

Since acne is a problem that does not affect overall health or life span, the simple fact that so many people seek treatment for it is revealing. Experts have long suspected, through the anecdotal evidence of those who suffer from acne, that it and other potentially disfiguring skin problems can cause feelings of insecurity and inferiority and can interfere in the way we live our day-to-day lives. Recent research has confirmed these intuitions.

A case of severe acne can cause problems such as a loss of self-confidence and social withdrawal. Studies have revealed that acne can interfere with our participation in social interactions such as sports and dating. Some people with acne suffer from lower levels of academic functioning, while others have higher rates of unemployment. Skin problems in general—and specifically acne—are not conditions to be taken lightly.

THE SYMPTOMS OF ACNE VULGARIS

The blemishes of acne can break out on the face, neck, back, and chest. Acne may first appear as one lone pimple, and then mushroom into a series of lesions such as *papules, pustules, comedones* (lesions that include *blackheads* and *whiteheads*), and *cysts*. The blemishes of acne include some combination of the following:

- Papules: Small bumps that may be red, white, or flesh-colored
- Pustules: Small bumps filled with pus
- Blackheads: Open comedones, which occur when follicles become clogged with dark, oily debris
- Whiteheads: Closed comedones, white papules, which are caused by a buildup of sebum that cannot penetrate the follicles
- Cysts: Closed sacs that contain some combination of the keratin scale, cellular debris, and oil gland secretions (These are the largest and most uncomfortable acne lesions, and the ones most likely to result in lasting scars.) Milia and hair follicle cysts are the two most common forms of cyst.

SELF-HELP FOR ACNE

Primary care for acne consists of practicing good hygiene and avoiding products that can aggravate acne-prone skin. Tips for treating acne include:

- Wash your face gently once or twice a day, using a mild soap or cleanser.
- Do not excessively wash or scrub your face, which can irritate skin and worsen acne.
- Use drying astringents with care, no more than once or twice a week.
- Shampoo your hair frequently, and make an effort to keep hair (if it is oily) off your face.
- Do not squeeze or pick at pimples; this may induce scarring.

- Avoid oil-based skin care products; use makeup that is water-based or oil-free.
- Choose skin care products that are labeled non-comedogenic—that is, products that are not likely to clog pores and cause the comedones (blackheads and whiteheads) that are typical of acne.
- Use flesh-tinted anti-blemish lotions (such as Clearasil or Rezamid) instead of cosmetics to cover acne.
- Use over-the-counter acne care products, which usually include some combination of the four major acne-fighting ingredients: benzoyl peroxide, resorcinol, salicylic acid, and sulfur. These products are available as creams, lotions, gels, and soaps.
- Avoid foods that are high in iodine—such as iodized salt, shellfish, and seaweed—which can trigger outbreaks of acne.
- Do *not* get a suntan to try to conceal acne. Due to damage from UVA rays and resultant clogging of pores, overexposure to the sun one day can lead to formation of whiteheads a month later. (Overuse of sunscreens can also clog pores and contribute to acne.)

If your acne does not respond to these measures, consult your dermatologist.

THE DERMATOLOGICAL TREATMENT OF ACNE

In some cases, inflammatory acne can become severe and, without dermatological intervention, can lead to deep scarring. Although early treatment of acne is best, your dermatologist can also help in cases where scarring has already occurred. Following are common preventive and post-scarring medical treatments that are available from your dermatologist:

Topical Anti-Acne Medications

In cases of mild to moderate acne, dermatologists usually prescribe topical medications. This strategy is designed to minimize the risk of potential side effects, which are associated more often with oral than with topical medications.

- **Retin-A** Retin-A—also known as tretinoin or retinoic acid—is a vitamin A derivative that may well be the most effective topical treatment for acne. Over time, Retin-A promotes healing of existing acne and prevents new eruptions from occurring. Retin-A has both keratolytic (peeling) and antimicrobial (germ-killing) qualities. It reduces cell turnover time and helps penetrate and loosen clogged pores.

  The most common forms of Retin-A are creams and gels, which must be used for three to four months for maximum benefit. A special advantage of Retin-A is that it increases the effectiveness of other topical agents and oral antibiotics when they are used in conjunction with it.

  Retin-A comes in various concentrations, but even low concentrations may leave skin dry, scaly, and red. To offset uncomfortable side effects, dermatologists usually prescribe a low dose to start out with and gradually increase it. Applying Retin-A to skin when it is dry may help minimize side effects. It's also especially important to avoid the sun or apply sunscreen during treatment, since Retin-A heightens your sensitivity to the sun.

- **Benzoyl Peroxide** Like Retin-A, benzoyl peroxide has keratolytic and antimicrobial qualities to aid in the penetration and loosening of clogged pores. Although benzoyl peroxide is not as potent as Retin-A, it is a valuable weapon against mild cases of acne.

  While benzoyl peroxide is available in over-the-counter acne remedies, your dermatologist can prescribe a higher concentration of benzoyl peroxide gel to improve acne lesions more rapidly and effectively. As with Retin-A, however, benzoyl peroxide can be drying to the skin. Therefore it's always a wise idea to begin with a lower concentration and use higher formulations only if the lower ones prove ineffective.

- **Topical Antibiotics**   Topical antibiotics can reduce acne lesions by 50 percent or more. The two most commonly prescribed and effective antibiotics for the topical management of moderate acne are *clindamycin* and *erythromycin*. Available as creams, lotions, and ointments, clindamycin and erythromycin should be applied sparingly to the skin. A little goes a long way, and overapplication can result in dry skin.

Selecting the Appropriate Topical Treatment for Acne

Selecting the right topical medication for your acne is important. Matters that you and your dermatologist will want to take into consideration include the nature of your acne lesions, any other medications you are taking, your complexion, and personal preference. Options include:

- **Creams**   Retin-A, benzoyl peroxide, and topical antibiotics are all available in cream formulations. Creams are a good choice for women who have sensitive skin. However, they may leave a slightly greasy residue.
- **Gels**   Retin-A, benzoyl peroxide, and topical antibiotics are all available in gel formulations. Gels leave no greasy residue, which makes them especially popular with women who have oily complexions. However, chemicals in gels may sting or burn skin that is traumatized or eczematous. In addition, cosmetics may not blend well into skin that has been treated with gel.

- **Lotions** Lotions are thinner than creams and are more compatible with cosmetic use than are gels. Lotions, which may contain Retin-A, benzoyl peroxide, or topical antibiotics, are a good choice for women who want to combine a moisturizer and acne treatment in one product.
- **Ointments** Few ointments are available for acne, since their greasy consistency is unappealing to most people. Still, topical antibiotic ointments may be an appropriate choice for older women with dry skin who also suffer from acne, and for teenagers who have both acne and eczema.
- **Solutions** Topical antibiotic solutions are a good choice for acne sufferers with very oily skin. Their astringent effect can replace regular use of a toner. Solutions should be avoided by women who have dry or sensitive skin.

Oral Anti-Acne Medications

Oral or systemic antibiotics, which subject your whole body to the effects of drugs, are seldom used before topical antibiotics are tried. But when topical therapies are not enough to get a severe case of acne under control, your dermatologist may prescribe oral anti-acne medications, notably *antibiotics* or *isotretinoin*. Isotretinoin, the oral form of retinoic acid, is the most powerful anti-acne medication available today. Oral medications have potent antibacterial and anti-inflammatory qualities which effectively reduce acne.

On the other hand, all these drugs must be taken for four to six months in order to be effective, and they have potentially serious side effects. These range from uncomfortable vaginal yeast infections and increased sun sensitivity, to a dangerous increase in the risk of birth defects in children of women who take isotretinoin. The risks versus the benefits of each oral medication must be carefully weighed before beginning any course of oral acne therapy.

ORAL ACNE MEDICATIONS: IMPORTANT CONCERNS FOR WOMEN

It is absolutely crucial that women of childbearing age discuss the possible side effects of oral acne medications with their dermatologists before proceeding with either of the following:

- **Tetracycline,** a common oral antibiotic, may *decrease* the effectiveness of oral contraceptives when it is taken over time. Always use alternative forms of birth control when you take tetracycline, or ask your dermatologist to prescribe a different oral medication. (In fact, all oral antibiotics may decrease the effectiveness of oral contraceptives.)
- **Isotretinoin** should *never* be used by women who are, may be, or are planning to become pregnant. Isotretinoin is a *teratogen*, which means that it can cause birth defects.

Dermatological Treatment Procedures for Acne

Scars resulting from acne may be improved by chemical peels or dermabrasion, two procedures that should be performed in your dermatologist's office under local anesthesia. A careful consultation with your dermatologist is always recommended before cosmetic procedures such as these are performed.

- **Chemical Peels** In chemical peels, a mild acid is used to burn off the surface layer of skin, thus eliminating superficial acne scars and evening out overall skin tone. There are three types of chemical peels: superficial, medium, and deep. Medium and deep peels are painful, complicated procedures. A light chemical peel has fewer side effects, but may still cause swelling, redness, and extreme sensitivity to the sun for months following treatment.

- **Dermabrasion** In dermabrasion, skin is frozen with a spray medication, and a high-speed rotary abrasive wheel—a medical tool that is basically the equivalent of a mini-sander—is used to remove the top layer of skin. Dermabrasion is generally a more effective treatment for deep scars left by acne. As in the case of chemical peels, it's best to minimize sun exposure for several months after dermabrasion.

DERMATITIS AND ECZEMA

Dermatitis and *eczema* are two broad, umbrella terms for noncontagious skin rashes. The terms are often used interchangeably. Generally speaking, we can think of dermatitis, eczema, and even rashes as meaning the same thing. These are all inflammatory skin conditions that can be red or red *and* wet.

Dermatitis literally means "inflammation of the skin." Neither dermatitis nor eczema is caused by germs, therefore neither is contagious. Yet dermatitis, in the strictest definition, can also refer to inflammations of the skin caused by infections. If we put a word before "dermatitis"—such as "contact"—we can get a more specific definition of its meaning. *Eczema,* on the other hand, no matter what adjectives may be attached to the term, refers to noncontagious rashes only.

In this chapter, we will focus on skin rashes that are not caused by germs and are not, therefore, contagious. Characteristics of these rashes frequently include swelling, itching, blistering, oozing, thickening, peeling, and scabbing. The two most common types of dermatitis are atopic and contact dermatitis.

WHAT IS ECZEMA?

Eczema refers to any noncontagious, inflammatory skin rash that may be caused by hypersensitivity or allergy. Eczema is often characterized by excruciating itching. Although many allergic people also have eczema, strictly speaking eczema is not an allergic reaction.

About a third to a half of all skin conditions can be classified as eczema. People who have long-standing wet rashes also tend to get secondary bacterial infections. In general, the following lesions are typical of eczema:

- Macules: nonelevated red skin spots
- Papules: small bumps that may be red, white, or flesh-colored
- Pustules: small white bumps filled with pus
- Vesicles: small fluid-filled blisters
- Scales and crusts: flaking, peeling layers of skin

ATOPIC DERMATITIS: CAUSES, SYMPTOMS, AND TREATMENT

Atopy is the inherited predisposition to become hypersensitive or allergic to substances such as pollen, ragweed, dust mites, molds, and animal scales or droppings. About 15 percent of the people in the United States are atopic, according to the American Academy of Dermatology. Two ways this condition manifests itself are through hives and through atopic dermatitis, which is also known as chronic eczema. (Other manifestations of atopy are asthma, hay fever, and migraine headaches.) Yet while most cases of atopic dermatitis are due to a genetic predisposition, it is also possible to develop this problem even if no one else in your family has suffered from it.

Dermatologists refer to atopic dermatitis as the itch that rashes; it is so itchy that it produces secondary rashes from scratching.

The symptoms of atopic dermatitis may begin in infancy and occur on and off throughout one's lifetime. Episodes of atopic dermatitis may be set off by emotional stress or physical injury, and people with the disorder usually have very dry and sensitive skin. In adults, skin may become thick and leathery and develop painful cracks.

The treatment of atopic dermatitis varies according to its severity. The regular use of moisturizers on dry, atopic skin is helpful. Atopy is almost always characterized by pruritis, or itching. It's also best for atopic individuals to take natural measures such as wearing cotton fabrics and keeping their homes, especially their bedrooms, free of potential irritants, such as dust and dust mites, animal dander, and molds. A combination of anti-inflammatory topical corticosteroids and oral antihistamines to relieve itching may be prescribed by your dermatologist to relieve chronic or severe rashes.

PRURITUS: THE MOST COMMON SYMPTOM IN DERMATOLOGY

Pruritus is the dermatological term for itching and covers the whole spectrum from a mild urge to scratch to an overwhelming and almost unbearable itch. Pruritus plays a major role in countless skin rashes, including eczema, psoriasis, and many forms of contact dermatitis. Eczema is almost always accompanied by very intense pruritus.

Cool water and ice can provide quick relief from itching. Frequent use of moisturizers and modifying your environment to add humidity are measures you can take to control itching. Oatmeal baths are also soothing. In serious cases of eczema, however, your dermatologist may recommend or prescribe medications to control pruritus.

CONTACT DERMATITIS: CAUSES, SYMPTOMS, AND TREATMENT

Contact dermatitis is an inflammatory response of the skin to a specific substance to which you have developed an allergy or sensitization. Unlike atopic dermatitis, contact dermatitis is not associated with genetic predisposition, nor is it triggered or worsened by stress or physical injury. Symptoms of contact dermatitis range from wet blistering to dry cracking and scaling of skin.

The primary treatment of contact dermatitis is the same as that of atopic dermatitis: identification and avoidance of triggers. Medical care, like that for atopic dermatitis, may include a combination of antihistamines to relieve itching and topical corticosteroids to combat local inflammation.

Two major types of contact dermatitis are allergic and irritant:

- **Allergic contact dermatitis** is caused by an allergic reaction, in which histamine is released from mast cells in the skin, causing itching, reddening, and inflammation. (An allergy is an overreaction or hypersensitivity developed to a substance that is harmless to most individuals. Allergic reactions do not occur the first time you come into contact with a particular substance, but may develop after repeated exposure to that substance.) An oozing and blistering red rash characterizes this type of dermatitis.

  Poison ivy, oak, and sumac are the classic examples of allergic contact dermatitis. Some people also develop allergies to nickel, which is commonly found in rings and other jewelry, tools, and appliances. Others are sensitive to the chemicals and fragrances used in cosmetics and perfumes.

- **Irritant contact dermatitis** is even more common than its allergic counterpart. Rashes ranging from mild to severe develop when your skin comes into contact with a primary irritant. A common example of irritant contact dermatitis is so-called hand eczema, which, in years gone by, was more frequently referred to as "housewives' eczema." This is a red, itchy rash often due to contact with harsh chemicals or irritants in soaps, detergents, and other cleansers.

However, irritant contact dermatitis is by no means limited to hands alone. This rash may develop wherever contact occurs. Modern processing of fabrics to make them waterproof or stain-resistant, chemicals used by dry cleaners, dyes, cosmetics, and perfumes are all potential triggers of irritant contact dermatitis.

HIVES

Hives—technically known as *urticaria* and commonly called *welts* or *wheals*—are irregular, round swellings brought on by an allergic reaction. Inflammation and extremely intense itching accompany hives. Bouts of uncomfortable hives can last from hours to days, and 20 percent of us will experience them at some point in our lifetime.

WHAT CAUSES HIVES?

Common causes of hives are allergic reactions to foods, drugs, and infections. A number of foods—such as nuts, berries, and shellfish—cause repeated episodes of hives, so it's best to identify these foods and eliminate them from your diet. Infections that can bring on hives include bacteria such as staphylococcus and streptococcus, chicken pox, mononucleosis, and vaginal yeast infections. Penicillin and penicillin-like drugs may also produce hives and should not be taken by people who are sensitive to them. Chronic hives—bouts that occur daily for more than three to six weeks—have been associated with atopy, eczema, infection, drugs, emotional stress, and extremes in temperature.

COMMON TRIGGERS OF HIVES

Although foods and drugs are not the only triggers of hives, they are the most common causes of this condition. Do not eat any food or take any drug that you and your physician suspect may be causing your hives. Here is a list of the most likely suspects:

- **Foods**
  Additives and preservatives
  Beans
  Chocolate
  Eggs
  Nuts
  Seasonings
  Shellfish
  Strawberries
  Tomatoes
- **Drugs**
  Aspirin
  Codeine
  Penicillin
  Sulfa drugs
  Tetracycline

THE SYMPTOMS OF HIVES

The local red swellings of hives may be as small as a pencil eraser, or many hives may join together to form a lesion as large as a plate. Acute urticaria are single attacks that last from hours to days, and chronic urticaria can last for weeks.

THE TREATMENT OF HIVES

The most effective treatment for hives is to discern their cause and eliminate it from your environment. In the meantime, antihistamines can relieve the uncomfortable, allergic symptoms of hives. Over-the-counter or prescription topical steroids can reduce hives. In very severe cases, short bursts of oral steroids may be given. Hot water should be avoided, since it excites hives and makes itching worse. Since all drugs have side effects, your best strategy is to pinpoint and avoid the triggers of hives.

PITYRIASIS ROSEA

Pityriasis rosea is a benign skin rash that often begins with a single pink patch on the chest or back and then spreads. The rash usually lasts for a period of weeks to months and disappears without leaving a scar. Those affected are usually between ten and thirty-five years of age.

WHAT CAUSES PITYRIASIS ROSEA?

The cause of pityriasis rosea remains unknown. Although it is currently classified as a noninfectious disease by the American Academy of Dermatology, more and more scientists today believe that pityriasis rosea is due to a virus. Until this has been proven, it will continue to be classified as noninfectious. Pityriasis rosea is not caused by a fungus or bacterial infection and does not appear to be an allergic reaction.

THE SYMPTOMS OF PITYRIASIS ROSEA

The initial scaly pink patch of pityriasis rosea is called the "mother" or "herald" patch. In a week or two smaller pink patches will spread from the mother patch over the trunk of the body, frequently in a distinctive pattern resembling a drooping evergreen tree. Itching accompanies some but not all cases, and there is occasional aching or tiredness. Most rashes fade after six weeks or so, while others persist for longer periods of time.

THE TREATMENT OF PITYRIASIS ROSEA

Pityriasis rosea is sometimes mistaken for ringworm (an itchy, red fungal rash in the shape of a ring) or a reaction to medications such as antibiotics. Your dermatologist will order tests such as skin scrapings or a biopsy to confirm the diagnosis of pityriasis rosea. A blood test is occasionally necessary as well to rule out contagious infections that may present similar rashes.

Treatment for mild cases of pityriasis rosea consists of the application of anti-itching lotions. In addition, hot baths and strenuous activity can irritate the rash and should be avoided. If these measures prove inadequate, your dermatologist may recommend ultraviolet light treatments or oral anti-inflammatory medications. When a physician prescribes ultraviolet therapy, it is through controlled doses and delivery, which reduces risk. Yet since side effects may be associated with these treatments, be sure to discuss their risks and benefits with your dermatologists.

PSORIASIS

As the top layer of your skin wears away, cells produced beneath the surface normally rise up to replace it. But in *psoriasis,* these new skin cells form too rapidly, then die and pile up faster than the skin can shed them. Consequently, the thick and unsightly lesions of psoriasis develop.

Psoriasis is a chronic, noncontagious skin disease characterized by red, scaly patches that are often extremely itchy. Widespread psoriasis can be disfiguring and, like acne, may cause emotional discomfort and embarrassment. In addition, serious cases of psoriasis may lead to painful cracking, or fissuring, of the skin. In a small number of instances, psoriatic arthritis (a painful form of arthritis affecting the fingers, toes, and spine) may precede or follow psoriasis of the skin.

WHAT CAUSES PSORIASIS?

Although the exact cause of psoriasis remains unknown, genetic predisposition is thought to play an important role. If a parent or close relative suffers from this condition, you are more likely to develop it.

Psoriasis can occur in varying degrees of severity throughout life, and flare-ups are linked to a variety of triggers, including emotional stress, hormonal changes, injuries to the skin, and overexposure to the sun.

SKIN DISORDERS AND STRESS

Skin disorders such as psoriasis and hives may be either brought on or aggravated by anxiety, tension, and emotional stress. Yet other factors— such as your own genetic predisposition, allergies, and any physical injury—usually play the most important roles in determining whether or not you develop skin rashes.

THE SYMPTOMS OF PSORIASIS

Psoriasis is characterized by raised red or pink lesions that are often covered by thick, silvery scales. The onset of psoriasis can be swift and severe, or gradual and mild. Lesions range from small patches of dandruff-like scaling to major eruptions covering large areas of skin.

Although psoriasis may affect any skin area, it most commonly appears on the scalp, elbows, knees, lower back, hands, feet, armpits, and genitals. The lesions ordinarily cause more emotional than physical upset; however, itching, cracking, bleeding, soreness and aching joints (in the case of psoriatic arthritis) may occur.

The manifestations of psoriasis range from mild to potentially life-threatening and equally affect women and men. Correct diagnosis is important, since while psoriasis may at times resemble eczema, the two are distinct and unrelated conditions. Fortunately, there are many treatments for psoriasis, although there is still no cure for the condition.

THE TREATMENT OF PSORIASIS

In order to properly diagnose psoriasis, your dermatologist may perform a biopsy on a small sample of your skin. This will distinguish psoriasis from seemingly similar diseases, such as eczema or fungal infections. Treatment then varies according to the relative severity of the condition.

Self-treatment alone is seldom recommended for psoriasis. For most people, treatment generally involves a combination of self-help and prescription medication. In mild cases of psoriasis, scales are softened with prescribed medications and then gently removed from the skin using a soft brush in an oatmeal bath. This must be done on a daily basis. Helpful over-the-counter products include coal-tar soaps, shampoos, and cleansers. Coal tar helps to reduce the thickness, redness, and itching of psoriasis lesions. It's also best to avoid scratching or picking at lesions, which may cause them to thicken.

In more serious cases of psoriasis, your dermatologist may prescribe stronger formulations of coal-tar or topical steroid preparations. In very severe cases, low doses of potent cytotoxic drugs, which are poisonous to cells, are given orally to slow cell division. And exposure to ultraviolet light (both UVA and UVB rays) is recommended in stubborn cases of psoriasis that do not respond to other forms of treatment. Again, prescription ultraviolet light is carefully controlled in both dosage and delivery by your physician, and this type of treatment will be used only when the benefits clearly outweigh the risks of UV exposure.

MANAGING SKIN PROBLEMS

In this chapter we have discussed the causes, symptoms, and treatment of the most common noninfectious rashes. Among their many manifestations is a range in discomfort from mild irritation to maddening itch. In the next chapter we will explore the broad range of forms that infectious skin diseases may take, and the most effective ways to manage them.

CHAPTER 6

Not surprisingly, as you've seen by now, the largest and most visible organ of your body is host to a multitude of diseases. Every year millions of people require medical treatment for newly diagnosed skin problems. In previous chapters we discussed skin cancer and noninfectious skin rashes. Here we'll examine how we manage other common skin difficulties, including infections, sexually transmitted diseases, and pigmentation and blood vessel problems.

VIRAL INFECTIONS

Among the most common viral skin infections are the sexually transmitted diseases genital herpes and genital warts. The viruses that cause these conditions are highly contagious and are spread through intimate sexual contact. Shingles, on the other hand, is caused by the varicella virus (a member of the herpes family of viruses), the same virus that causes chicken pox in children. Stress and weakened immune systems may reactivate this dormant virus in people who had chicken pox as children.

HERPES SIMPLEX

Herpes simplex is the most common sexually transmitted disease, with an estimated 80 percent of the adult population carrying a form of the virus. The herpes simplex virus causes cold sores and fever blisters around the mouth, and genital sores known as genital herpes.

There are two herpes simplex viruses: herpes simplex type 1 (HSV-1) and herpes simplex type 2 (HSV-2). The viruses are similar, and both can infect either the mouth or genitals. But more commonly, HSV-1 is responsible for sores of the mouth, while HSV-2 causes genital sores.

What Causes Herpes Simplex?

Herpes simplex is caused by one of the two HSV viruses. The infection is spread through direct skin-to-skin contact, most often—although not exclusively—when an active infection is present. If you have a cold sore, for example, kissing someone may pass the virus on to them. In the case of active genital herpes, any type of direct sexual contact can transfer the virus from one person to another. In many cases, however, the herpes virus can be transmitted when there are no symptoms present; or it can be spread by people who don't even know they are infected. These individuals are known as silent carriers.

The Symptoms of Herpes Simplex

The symptoms of herpes simplex vary from person to person. A herpes attack evolves over a three- to five-day period. Early warning signs or so-called prodromal symptoms of a herpes outbreak may include burning, stinging, tingling, itching, and tenderness at the site of the outbreak. Eventually a red bump develops, which evolves over time into a blister and then into a pustule. Pustules are sometimes mistaken for impetigo, a common and very contagious bacterial skin infection.

- **The First Episode of Herpes** After intimate contact with a person infected with the virus, herpes symptoms usually develop within two to twenty days. At the beginning of infection, the herpes virus bypasses the immune system defenses by entering nerve endings. In some people, the first herpes attack may be quite mild. In others, the first attack is accompanied by visible sores.

The typical symptoms of the first episode of herpes include inflamed skin that soon forms blisters. Blisters open and then heal as new skin tissue develops. The affected area often itches and burns. Flu-like symptoms, such as fever, aches, headache, and swollen glands may accompany the first episode of herpes simplex.

- **Recurrent Episodes of Herpes** Once you have herpes, you have it for life. In fact, 80 to 90 percent of people who have genital herpes have recurrent outbreaks. Some people have frequent recurrences, while others have few. The average number of recurrences of genital herpes is four per year, although this number decreases over time.

  The herpes virus lies dormant in your nervous system until triggered by such factors as stress, fatigue, illness, surgery, diet, menstruation, sexual activity, or skin irritation (such as sunburn). When prodromal symptoms such as tingling and itching occur, preceding the actual onset of skin sores, herpes is already contagious.

  Fortunately, because the body develops antibodies to the herpes virus during the first episode, your immune system is better prepared to fight off infection in subsequent episodes. As a result, recurrences usually involve fewer sores, which heal more quickly.

The Treatment of Herpes Simplex

Although there is no cure for herpes, the prescription medicine oral acyclovir has proven to be effective in reducing the number and severity of herpes infections. Keeping the infected area clean and dry will also help clear up the outbreak, and you should avoid wearing garments that fit too tightly if you suffer from genital herpes. A balanced diet, exercise, and rest will boost your immune system, which may help keep the virus under control.

HERPES ZOSTER (SHINGLES)

Herpes zoster, or shingles, is an uncomfortable outbreak of skin sores that occurs in adults who have had chicken pox earlier in life.

What Causes Shingles?

Both chicken pox and shingles are caused by the same virus: varicella, a member of the herpes family. The first infection with the varicella virus is chicken pox. After the initial chicken pox infection, the virus remains dormant in the body, resting in nerve cells near the spinal cord and other organs. The virus is harmless until it is reactivated by factors such as physical or emotional stress or possibly through the natural weakening of the immune system as we age. Once reactivated, the varicella virus travels along the nerves to the skin and causes shingles.

The Symptoms of Shingles

Shingles is a painful eruption of many tiny, fluid-filled blisters on a reddish base, which may over time evolve to pustules. Early signs of a shingles outbreak often include numbness, tingling, or shooting pains in the nerve roots of linear areas, such as the arms, legs, and trunk of the body. A rash of blisters may then emerge in a bandlike pattern over the affected nerve or nerves, usually on one side of the body, back, or face. Flu-like symptoms such as fever, headache, and stomachache frequently accompany shingles.

The manifestations of shingles range from mild to severe. In some people, sores resemble the original lesions of chicken pox. In others, the pain of shingles interferes with the ordinary activities of daily life. Pustules that are initially clear turn cloudy as white blood cells attack the virus and eventually crust over, scab, and heal.

Unfortunately, even after blisters heal, many people continue to experience pain due to inflammation of the underlying nerves. People over sixty are apt to have subsequent nerve pain, or neuralgia, for months or even years after a case of shingles.

The Treatment of Shingles

There is no cure for shingles, but treatments are available. The prescription medication oral acyclovir was formerly the most effective antiviral medication for shingles, since it specifically attacks the varicella virus inside infected nerve cells. Acyclovir prevents the virus from replicating, helping to stop new blisters from forming and enabling existing blisters to heal more rapidly. This drug is most effective when used within the first few days of a shingles rash.

Yet a major new development in the treatment of shingles has been the introduction of the new antiviral drug, valaciclovir. Valaciclovir, which is rapidly converted into acyclovir after oral administration, attacks the varicella virus more quickly than acyclovir, providing faster and more efficient pain relief for shingles sufferers.

WARTS

Warts are caused by the human papilloma virus, or HPV, of which there are over one hundred different types. Flat warts on body areas such as the face, hands, and neck may be cosmetically unappealing. And while many warts are disfiguring, warts in sensitive areas (such as plantar warts, on the soles of the feet) can also be quite painful. The presence of many warts on your body may indicate that there is an underlying problem in the immune system.

What Causes Warts?

The human papilloma virus ordinarily enters the body through small cuts or abrasions and causes warts. HPVs can remain dormant in your skin cells for years, possibly causing additional warts in the future.

The Symptoms of Warts

Some HPVs grow and thrive on the soles of the foot (plantar warts) while others appear on the hands (palmar warts) or around the fingernails (periungual warts). Plantar warts are usually flat and calloused, while warts on the hands and around the fingernail are raised. Warts on the neck and face are smooth and flat.

The Treatment of Warts

At this moment there is no specific antiviral remedy for warts, and treatment should be aimed at decreasing discomfort and avoiding scarring. Over-the-counter treatments may be effective for those who have minor warts on the hands or feet, and many warts clear up without treatment. Dermatological procedures to remove warts include:

- **Application of chemicals or chemical compounds,** such as podofilox, podophyllin, and trichloracetic acid, to the surface of the wart
- **Curettage,** a procedure in which warts are scooped out with a sharp, spoon-shaped instrument called a curette (Success rates vary.)
- **Cryotherapy,** freezing off warts with liquid nitrogen (A number of cryotherapy treatments are usually necessary.)

- **Electrocautery,** the destruction of infected tissue with electric current (one of the most successful ways to remove warts and prevent them from recurring).
- **Laser therapy,** the use of an intense light to destroy warts (Special air ventilators are required as lasers airize the virus.)

GENITAL WARTS

Genital warts is one of the most common sexually transmitted diseases in the United States. As many as one million cases of genital warts are diagnosed every year. Warts on other parts of the body—most commonly on the hands and feet—are caused by different types of the human papilloma virus, or HPV, and contact with these warts is not thought to cause genital warts.

What Causes Genital Warts?

Genital warts are caused by the human papilloma virus, or genital HPV. There are thought to be more than one hundred different types of HPVs. Some cause warts on the hands or feet, while others cause genital warts. Genital warts are spread through intimate skin-to-skin contact.

The Symptoms of Genital Warts

Genital warts appear in the genital region and may be flat or raised, painless or itchy, single or multiple. Some form cauliflower-like clusters. Sometimes warts are inside the vagina and are not noticeable, so it is possible to have genital HPV and not know it. Because of this, it is vitally important to have regular Pap smears once you become sexually active.

The Treatment of Genital Warts

Health care providers generally discover genital warts through physical exams. In some women, they may be detected through abnormal Pap smears. You should visit your doctor if you notice any unusual growths, bleeding, itching, or pain in the genital area, or if your sexual partner has genital warts. Wart lesions may also be secondary to syphilis.

Over-the-counter treatments are meant for warts on hands and feet—*not* for warts in the sensitive genital area. Medical treatment of genital warts varies, and many doctors advise abstention from sex while warts heal. Common treatment options are the same as those used on other types of warts (see page 101).

GENITAL WARTS AND HERPES ARE ASSOCIATED WITH AN INCREASED RISK OF CERVICAL CANCER

Women who are sexually active are at a greater risk of sexually transmitted diseases, including genital warts and herpes, which have been linked to cervical cancer. If you are sexually active, you should protect yourself through the use of latex condoms and spermicide. In addition, you should be monitored frequently by your doctor. It's important to get a Pap smear every six months to a year, as cervical abnormalities that may indicate cancer are frequently detected through Pap smears.

SEXUALLY TRANSMITTED DISEASES AND YOUR SKIN

Sexually transmitted diseases (STDs) loom large in the world of skin problems. An estimated 10 to 12 million Americans have STDs. Sores, bumps, or blisters near the sex organs, rectum, or mouth are a frequent signs of sexually transmitted diseases. If a person has one STD, such as the most common STD herpes, it is likely that he or she has other STDs as well.

Anyone who is sexually active, regardless of age, race, socio-economic status, or sexual preference, can be infected with highly contagious STDs. Transmission of most STDs takes place only through intimate contact with an infected person, since the organisms that cause most STDs die quickly when removed from the human body.

Whereas syphilis and gonorrhea were once the most wide-spread STDs, today these diseases are largely under control, and diseases such as herpes and chlamydia are far more common. HIV infection is also on the rise. If you suspect that you have a sexually transmitted disease, see your doctor. Local exams, smears, cultures, biopsies, and blood tests are diagnostic tests your doctor may use to determine the nature of your problem.

If you do have an STD, you and your sexual partner should both be treated. STDs are asymptomatic in some individuals, and couples can easily pass diseases back and forth to one another. Pregnant women should notify their doctors if they have an active STD or have experienced an STD such as herpes in the past, since sexually transmitted diseases may cause difficulties during pregnancy or be passed on to babies.

STDs, formerly known as veneral diseases, are often caused by the viruses mentioned in the above section. Other common STDs include:

- **Candida vaginitis** Candida—also known as monili-asis—is a common and highly contagious yeast infection that causes redness and swelling in the genital area. Candida in women is characterized by intense itching and a cheesy white discharge, and may lead to painful erosive vulvitis. Over-the-counter antifungal agents are topically applied to cure candida, while prescription oral antifungal agents can cure more resistant infections. In some cases, a specific antiyeast ointment such as Lotrimin may be prescribed.

- **Chancroid** Chancroid is characterized by foul-smelling, pus-covered genital sores. It is caused by the bacteria Hemophilus ducreyi, diagnosed by culture, and is cured through treatment with prescription antibiotics such as oral erythromycin.

- **Chlamydia** Chlamydia, one of the more common STDs today, is caused by the bacterium Chlamydia trachomatis. Left untreated, chlamydia is a major cause of pelvic inflammatory disease (PID) and infertility in women. Chlamydia is diagnosed by culture and cured with appropriate prescription antibiotics. Recurrent or persistent chlamydia may be a warning sign of a serious medical infection. It is important to see your doctor for a complete evaluation.

- **Gonorrhea** Gonorrhea is caused by a bacteria that grows in the genital area or the throat. While 75 percent of women are asymptomatic, some women may experience symptoms such as a cloudy vaginal discharge, abdominal and back pain, and a sore throat. The diagnosis of gonorrhea is made through smears and cultures and it can be successfully treated with prescription antibiotics. Left untreated, gonorrhea can lead to pelvic inflammatory disease.

- **Hepatitis B** Hepatitis B is a common sexually transmitted viral disease. People can be infected without knowing and become carriers of the disease, capable of transmitting hepatitis B to others and at risk themselves for developing potentially fatal liver disease. Treatment consists of the use of prescription hepatitis B immune globulin (HBIG) combined with the hepatitis B vaccine.

- **HIV Infection and AIDS**   HIV (human immunodeficiency virus) infection and AIDS (Acquired Immunodeficiency Syndrome) manifest themselves in a variety of skin conditions, including many of the sexually transmitted diseases discussed in this chapter. More women are being infected with the HIV virus today than ever before, and the infection progresses more rapidly in women. HIV infection and AIDS, which are most commonly transmitted through intimate sexual contact and shared needles, leave the immune system weakened and the body vulnerable to a number of opportunistic diseases. Presently there is no cure for AIDS, but a variety of drugs makes it possible to live longer with HIV infection and AIDS.
- **Lice and Scabies**   Lice and scabies are parasitic infestations of the genital area that cause *profound* itching. Lice move from hair to hair like crabs, while scabies are buried in the skin. Parasitic infections were once looked down upon as diseases of lower socioeconomic groups. Today we know that these infestations—like other STDs—make no such distinctions. These uncomfortable, itchy rashes may be treated with lotions such as over-the-counter RID or prescription Kwell, which contain powerful pesticides. While lice are visible to the naked eye, people should not try to diagnose scabies themselves. The diagnosis may be easily missed. Proper treatment of lice and scabies infections depends upon severity, with more severe cases requiring prescription treatments from your dermatologist.
- **Molluscum contagiosum**   Molluscum contagiosum is a contagious viral disease that causes whitish bumps with red dimpled centers in the genital area. It is caused by the poxvirus. Treatment is the same as for genital warts.

- **Syphilis** Syphilis is a highly contagious disease caused by organisms known as spirochetes. The incubation time after infection is one to three months, during which time syphilis is already contagious. In the early stages of syphilis painless button-like papules appear at the site of infection, and later swollen lymph nodes develop. Syphilis can be cured through the administration of prescription penicillin antibiotics. Left untreated, syphilis can lead to serious and sometimes fatal complications, including heart disease, paralysis, insanity, and blindness.
- **Trichomoniasis** Trichomoniasis, or "trich," is caused by a one-celled parasitic organism known as a protozoan. It is characterized by burning, itching, and a thick, cream-colored vaginal discharge. Lower abdominal pain may also be present. Treatment consists of prescription antimicrobial medication, especially Flagyl.

ARE GENITAL DEODORANTS APPROPRIATE?

Practicing routine genital hygiene and avoiding tight clothing that can irritate skin should preclude the necessity of genital deodorants for most women. The skin in your groin area is as thin and delicate as that of your mucous membranes, and you are apt to do more harm than good by applying genital deodorants.

A foul-smelling vaginal discharge is the sign of a number of vaginal infections, including candida, chlamydia, and trichomoniasis. If you experience this symptom, see your gynecologist. Genital deodorants are *not* the answer to this problem and can seriously aggravate the condition.

HOW TO AVOID SEXUALLY TRANSMITTED DISEASES

Certain basic rules apply to reducing or eliminating your risk of sexually transmitted diseases:

- Abstain from sex.
- Have sex with only one noninfected partner, who also only has sex with you.
- Use condoms and spermicides when you are unsure whether you or your partner are free of infection.
- If sexually active, get yourself checked every six months to a year.

FUNGAL INFECTIONS

Many harmless fungi, in company with other microorganisms, commonly live on your skin. Fungi are microscopic plants—with leaves, stems, and seeds or spores—that grow on your skin. Usually these mold- or yeastlike organisms live in balance with your skin, feasting on sebum and scales. But under certain circumstances, such as when your immune system is weakened by physical disease or emotional stress, fungi grow out of control and cause infections on the skin. Usually doctors can eliminate the leaves and stems of fungi through treatment, but spores, which may be buried in the skin, can grow up again.

Fungi present a wide array of symptoms. Most fungal infections are characterized by itchy, scaly, peeling patches or round lesions, which are often mistaken for eczema or psoriasis. Skin condition ranges from slightly beige and scaly patches to pimply, large-scale erosions. Diagnosis depends on close examination of skin scrapings under a microscope; fungal infections are identified by slender filaments known as *hyphae*. Depending on the severity of fungal infections, either topical or oral antifungal medications—or some combination of the two—will be recommended by your dermatologist. Secondary bacterial infections are treated with antibiotics.

RINGWORM

Ringworm is not caused by a worm at all; it is caused by a fungus. Yet ringworm is very aptly named, since it produces an itchy, red rash in the shape of a ring. Ringworm is most often seen on the arms, legs, chest, and back. Once your doctor has identified the problem as ringworm, a topical antifungal medication can be used to cure the condition. Occasionally, prescription oral antifungals must be used.

ATHLETE'S FOOT

Athlete's foot, or tinea pedis, is characterized by itchy, scaly, flaking round patches or lesions between the toes (toe webs) or on the soles of feet. The color of patches may be red, grayish, or white. Athletic activity may induce sweating, which can bring on athlete's foot.

Diagnosis is made by skin scrapings and culture and is up to your dermatologist, since athlete's foot may be easily confused with eczema, psoriasis, or allergic contact dermatitis to shoes or socks. Treatment varies according to the degree of severity. Many effective over-the-counter topical, and new prescription oral antifungal medications are available. Prescription oral antibiotics may also be required when acute infections involve blistering, pustules, or oozing, as when you develop an allergic or immune response.

"JOCK ITCH"

Tinea cruris, more commonly known as "jock itch," is usually associated with men, but jock itch is a problem that affects women as well. This burning, itchy rash in the groin area usually occurs when moisture and heat are trapped close to the skin by underwear or pantyhose. You can fend off a case of tinea cruris by keeping the genital area dry and clean; helpful strategies include using talc and wearing cotton garments that breathe. Treatment consists of the application of antifungal medications. In severe cases, you may need to see your doctor for blood tests to eliminate the possibility of more serious underlying infections.

HOW TO AVOID FUNGAL INFECTIONS

- Keep skin cool and dry with proper after shower and bath care. Pay special attention to skin areas susceptible to fungal infection.
- Wear natural fabrics, such as cotton, that can "breathe."
- Avoid synthetic fibers, which do not absorb moisture well.
- Do not share hats, combs, or brushes.
- Change socks whenever your feet become sweaty.
- Frequently launder socks, towels, athletic supporters, and bath mats.
- Avoid close contact with infected persons or pets, since fungal infections are highly contagious.

BACTERIAL INFECTIONS

Bacterial skin infections, or pyodermas, are usually caused by one of two organisms, staphylococci ("staph") or streptococci ("strep"). Diagnosing bacterial infections is usually a simple process of identifying characteristic lesions. A culture test is often performed as well to confirm the type of bacterial organisms responsible for the infection, in order to choose the antibiotic best suited to eliminate them. Depending on the severity of bacterial infections, either topical or oral antibiotics—or some combination of the two—will be recommended by your doctor.

IMPETIGO

Impetigo, the most common bacterial skin infection, is usually caused by group A staphylococci. While impetigo commonly affects children, it is often brought home from day care centers and schools and passed on to adults. The disease can be spread through direct contact with infected persons or by touching articles that have been handled by infected persons.

Impetigo is characterized by pus-filled blisters that erupt and harden to form yellow crusts from which fluid may ooze. Impetigo may cause intense itching. Exposed parts of the skin—such as the face, hands, arms, and legs—may first fall victim to impetigo, but scratching blisters will cause it to spread to adjacent body areas.

The treatment of impetigo usually consists of gently removing yellow crusts with mild soap and water, and applying antibiotic ointment to affected areas. If impetigo is severe, oral antibiotics are often necessary. When promptly diagnosed and treated, the infection usually disappears within a week, and does not leave lasting scars.

FOLLICULITIS

Folliculitis, an inflammation of the hair follicles or pores, is usually caused by staphyloccal bacteria. Often mistaken for acne, it is characterized by many small red bumps (papules) or pus bumps (pustules) in the hair follicle openings where the hair meets the skin. Folliculitis occurs when bacteria and cell debris clog the hair follicle. Many women refer to folliculitis as "razor bumps," since it commonly occurs on the legs and in the bikini area due to the repeated trauma of shaving. Treatment of folliculitis consists of a combination of prescription topical and oral antibiotics.

FURUNCLES

Furuncles, more commonly known as boils, occur when bacteria penetrate follicles more deeply, causing severe inflammation of the surrounding skin. Furuncles are very contagious. Painful red boils, hot and tender to the touch, may be mistaken for the inflamed pimples of acne. Boils most often develop on the face, scalp, buttocks, or underarms.

Boils are potentially serious and should be treated by your doctor. Do not squeeze them or pick at them, as this may result in the spread of infection. When boils come to a head, your doctor may lance them. A preferred treatment is the application of over-the-counter and prescription antimicrobial and antiseptic agents and prescription oral antibiotics.

CARBUNCLES

One step beyond furuncles in degree of severity are carbuncles. Carbuncles, filled with bacteria, pus, and cell debris, are larger and deeper than boils. They also involve more hair follicles and surrounding tissue, and like furuncles are extremely contagious.

Carbuncles, like furuncles, can be a very serious condition if not diagnosed and treated promptly. Again, self-treatments such as squeezing or picking are counterproductive, as they may serve only to further spread infection. Your doctor may lance carbuncles when they come to a head, but the preferred treatment is oral antibiotics.

CELLULITIS

Cellulitis, an inflammatory condition that most commonly affects the legs, is usually caused by streptococci bacteria. This is a serious infection, often accompanied even in its early stages by a high fever, chills, and general weakness. Fortunately, like carbuncles, cellulitis usually responds well to an oral course of antibiotics; doctors often prescribe topical antibiotics to supplement oral therapy.

HYPERPIGMENTATION PROBLEMS

Hyperpigmentation is a common and usually benign condition in which patches of skin become darker than the color of normal surrounding skin. Hyperpigmentation can occur in people of any race. Common types of hyperpigmentation include age spots, melasma, and freckles.

WHAT CAUSES HYPERPIGMENTATION?

Darkening of the skin occurs due to an excess production of melanin (the brown pigmentation of the skin). Excess production may in turn be due to overexposure to the sun, hormonal changes, injury to the skin from disease or surgery, or genetic predisposition. Drugs such as birth control pills and hormone replacement therapy simulate hormones and can lead to hyperpigmentation.

Hyperpigmentation can grow more pronounced with increased sun exposure. This happens as melanin in existing patches absorbs the energy of the harmful ultraviolet rays of the sun in order to protect the skin from overexposure.

THE SIGNS OF HYPERPIGMENTATION

Hyperpigmentation manifests itself as age spots, freckles, and melasma:

- **Age spots,** also known as liver spots, frequently appear on the face, hands, back, and feet. Dermatologists refer to these flat, brown patches as solar lentigines. Age spots are primarily due to cumulative overexposure to the sun.

- **Freckles** are small brown spots that commonly appear on the face and arms. They are a harmless, inherited characteristic, but they can also be representative of sun damage.
- **Melasma,** or "the mask of pregnancy," is a darkening of pigmentation on facial skin during pregnancy due to some combination of hormonal changes, exposure to the sun, and genetic factors. Women who take birth control pills or hormone replacement therapy may also develop hyperpigmentation, since their bodies undergo hormonal changes similar to those in pregnancy. Melasma is most common on sun-exposed areas such as the face.

THE TREATMENT OF HYPERPIGMENTATION

In some cases, dark patches fade on their own. After giving birth, for example, many women find that hyperpigmentation gradually disappears. Avoidance of the sun is most important. And when you are exposed to the sun, be sure to use sunscreen.

Many women find freckles and age spots easy to live with, while others may turn to cosmetic concealers or skin bleach. Skin bleaches slow the production of melanin, so dark spots gradually fade to match normal surrounding skin. Both over-the-counter and stronger prescription skin bleaches are available.

VITILIGO: A CONDITION OF HYPOPIGMENTATION

Vitiligo is a kind of hypopigmentation, which is the opposite of hyperpigmentation. In this condition, for reasons which remain unknown, patches of skin become depigmented, as if bleach had been applied to them. Melanocytes are killed and therefore no more melanin or pigment is produced. The entertainer Michael Jackson is probably the best-known victim of vitiligo, a condition that can occur in people of all races and that affects women more commonly than men.

Camouflage makeup, when matched to skin tone and evenly applied, can cover the faded spots characteristic of vitiligo. Camouflage makeup is an opaque cosmetic product, in contrast to regular foundations, which are translucent and cannot cover blemishes. Medical treatments of vitiligo include the use of prescription topical and oral steroids, and PUVA therapy (psoralen drugs and exposure to controlled amounts of UVA light to repigment skin). When there is extensive damage, bleaching is also an alternative.

ROSACEA: A BLOOD VESSEL DISORDER

Rosacea is a vascular skin disease characterized by varying degrees of facial redness and thin red lines, due to the enlargement and dilation of blood vessels beneath the skin's surface. As redness progresses, pimples may also appear, which has often led to rosacea being mislabeled as acne. Yet though rosacea may include any of the acne-like lesions, acne and rosacea are two distinct skin conditions.

WHAT CAUSES ROSACEA?

The cause of rosacea is probably an infectious agent. Theories suggest that it may be caused by a type of yeast called pityrosporum, bacteria, a fungus, mites, a malfunction of connective tissues in the skin, or psychological factors. Yet none of these theories has been proven. Most likely, rosacea is due to some combination of factors in susceptible individuals. Susceptibility, in turn, may be affected by heredity, skin color, and skin structure.

Rosacea is most common in fair-skinned people; a Celtic ancestry may predispose one to rosacea, while blacks are rarely affected by the condition. Rosacea is most likely to develop in those over twenty years old and affects more women than men. But men who have rosacea are more likely to develop rhinophyma, or a puffy, swollen, red nose.

Although the cause of rosacea remains a mystery, the drinking of hot beverages, the consumption of caffeine and alcohol, and exposure to the sun and other forms of ultraviolet light have all been identified as potential triggers of rosacea because they precipitate flushing, which may aggravate the condition.

THE SYMPTOMS OF ROSACEA

Rosacea is a long-term disorder, characterized by periodic flare-ups that may worsen over time. The first sign of rosacea is usually a persistent redness on the face that may seem like a blush or sunburn. The symptoms of rosacea include some combination of the following:

- A persistent redness of the face, especially across the cheeks and nose
- Pimples (papules and/or pustules)
- Thin red lines called telangiectasia
- A puffy, swollen, red nose, or rhinophyma, a condition that is especially common in men who have rosacea (such as the late comedian W. C. Fields)

THE TREATMENT OF ROSACEA

Although there is no cure for rosacea, treatments are available to control rosacea and to improve skin appearance. Early medical intervention is best, since available care can halt the progression of rosacea. Self-treatment of the condition may backfire and is generally discouraged by dermatologists; over-the-counter acne medications, for example, may irritate the dry and sensitive skin of those who have rosacea.

If you have rosacea, one simple measure you can take is to identify and avoid factors that may trigger your flare-ups. These often include exposure to sunlight, extremes of heat and cold, stress, hot liquids, spicy foods, and alcohol. In general, it's best to steer clear of substances or actions that cause facial flushing.

Each case of rosacea is unique, and only your dermatologist can determine the treatment that is right for you. Medical recommendations for rosacea include the use of:

- Topical antimicrobial agents
- Oral antibacterial agents
- Topical steroids
- Mild soaps and cleansers
- Moisturizer
- Sunscreen

SEBORRHEIC DERMATITIS

Seborrheic dermatitis is a common and chronic skin rash characterized by redness and scaling. It occurs in the areas of skin where the sebaceous or oil glands are most active, such as scalp, the eyebrows, eyelashes, the middle of the face, the chest, and in skin or body folds.

WHAT CAUSES SEBORRHEIC DERMATITIS?

You may develop seborrheic dermatitis if you have a genetic predisposition to this condition. The yeast pityrosporum ovale may play a role in seborrheic dermatitis, as can a high fat diet and alcohol ingestion.

THE SYMPTOMS OF SEBORRHEIC DERMATITIS

Seborrheic dermatitis is most common in the triangle in the middle of the face. Redness and scaling are common. Seborrheic dermatitis of the scalp can lead to shedding of scalp hair.

THE TREATMENT OF SEBORRHEIC DERMATITIS

Seborrheic dermatitis is diagnosed through the examination of skin scrapings. New AHA astringents and hydrocortisone cream are used to treat facial seborrheic dermatitis. Seborrheic dermatitis of the scalp is treated with over-the-counter or prescription shampoos, depending on the severity of the problem.

FROM SKIN PROBLEMS TO SKIN CARE PRODUCTS

In the past several chapters we have seen that skin diseases are a widespread problem. Whereas some are benign, others can be serious and even life-threatening. Fortunately, there are many ways to prevent or treat skin disorders. Next we will explore how to determine your skin type and the most appropriate products you can use to keep your skin healthy and problem-free.

CHAPTER 7

The cosmetics industry is a more than 80 billion-dollar industry, and many a woman has strolled into a department store to buy a moisturizer only to be confronted with a bewildering and expensive array of merchandise. An astonishing collection of skin care products lines the shelves of drugstores, department stores, makeup salons, and spas, and products that are available range from the essential to the frivolous.

Yet today's women have full schedules, jam-packed with activities ranging from corporate board meetings to PTA meetings. Although we all want to have healthy skin and look and feel our best, our busy lifestyles simply cannot accommodate the complicated beauty regimes of yesteryear. So how do you choose the skin care products that are right for you?

Today's back-to-basics approach to healthy skin begins with a simple three-step process: cleanse, moisturize, and protect. You can take it from there, adding optional special treatments such as masks, toners, and makeup, as needed or desired. Every woman can develop a streamlined skin care process especially suited to meet her own individual requirements.

UNDERSTANDING YOUR SKIN TYPE

Skin care products are specifically formulated to care for and complement a variety of skin types, so the first step in choosing the right skin care products is to determine what type of skin you have: normal, dry, oily, or combination. Many women then have additional cosmetic priorities, such as highlighting attractive features and concealing flaws.

WHAT IS YOUR SKIN TYPE?

The women and men who staff cosmetics counters today often don white coats, consult computers, and administer skin tests to customers in a simulation of clinical efficiency. Yet it is usually just as easy, definitely less expensive, and often even more accurate to conduct your own skin test at home. Try this simple examination in the privacy of your home, alone or with a friend, to determine your skin type:

Wash your face and do not apply any skin product to it for the following hour. Then press a tissue to your forehead, cheeks, chin, and nose:

- If there's no oily residue on the tissue, you have normal skin.
- If skin particles appear on the tissue, you have dry skin. Flaking may also be evident on your skin. (If dry skin does not improve after moisturizing, you may have dermatitis and should see your doctor.)
- If all areas reveal oily residue, you have oily skin.
- If some areas of your skin leave an oily residue while others do not, you have combination skin.

SPECIAL SKIN CARE CONCERNS FOR DARK-SKINNED WOMEN

Today more and more women of color are choosing skin care products from product lines that are specially designed for a variety of dark skin shades and types. These products range from makeup to moisturizers to sunscreen. The more melanin you have in your skin, the darker your skin color. Melanin offers natural protection from the harmful ultraviolet rays of the sun, resulting in far fewer skin cancers in dark-skinned women. Because of this natural form of protection, dark-skinned women also appear to age more slowly than women who have fair skin. Wrinkles may not appear prominently on deeply pigmented skin until around the age of sixty, while white women in their forties are already contending with laugh lines and crows-feet.

All woman should use sunscreen with an SPF of at least 15. The appropriate SPF depends on the degree of melanin in your skin. A light-skinned black woman, for example, requires the same amount of sun protection as an olive-skinned white woman. A lower SPF is sufficient for black women with darker skin, while an albino black woman requires a higher Sun Protection Factor.

Skin problems unique to dark-skinned women often result from the use of heavy emollients to reduce ashy gray tones. Ashiness is due to dead, scaling cells on the surface of *dry* black skin—yet this is a case in which the "cure" is sometimes worse than the "disease." Many dark-skinned women use overly heavy moisturizers to reduce ashiness—but this often results in clogged pores, which in turn can lead to folliculitis and acne. Your best bet is to choose a moisturizer that is light, oil-free, and non-comedogenic but still effectively relieves dryness and corrects ashy tones.

THE THREE-STEP PROGRAM: CLEANSER, MOISTURIZER, AND SUNSCREEN

Today's streamlined approach to skin care emphasizes the use of three basic products: cleanser, moisturizer, and sunscreen.

The current philosophy is, Less Is Better. As we mentioned earlier, you can then build on this basic skin care routine, adding whatever additional products you feel are right for you. Extra-deep moisturizers, for example, may be appropriate for very dry skin. Skin that is very oily or acne-prone can benefit from the use of astringents or toners, which remove oily residue.

Combination products abound in this current environment where shortcuts to skin care are of the essence. Combinations offer two or more forms of convenient skin care in one easy step. Many gentle cleansers are enriched with moisturizers, while a number of moisturizers also offer protection from the harmful ultraviolet rays of the sun. And sunscreens often do double duty as moisturizers.

The three-step program of skin care is, of course, best for people who don't have a lot of skin problems. Additional steps must be added for those who have extra dry or oily skin. And, if you suffer from acute or chronic skin disorders such as acne, eczema, or rosacea, it is best to consult your dermatologist for help in devising an appropriate skin care program.

ARE COMBINATION PRODUCTS RIGHT FOR YOU?

A word of caution: It's important to choose the combination products that are right for you and to avoid those that may be either too much or not enough of a good thing. If you are using a moisturizer that also offers sun protection, for example, keep in mind that it is not necessary to have sunscreen on when you go to sleep at night. Conversely, if you simply apply a moisturizer with an SPF of 8 and cruise out for a day of sun and fun at the beach, your protection from harmful UV rays is woefully inadequate.

CLEANSER

The first step toward healthy skin is to wash your face once or twice a day with a mild cleanser. Cleansers are designed to remove oily residue, dead skin cells, dirt, and makeup, and products available today can cleanse thoroughly without stripping skin of natural protective oils. After cleansing, skin should always be thoroughly rinsed with lukewarm water; avoid using hot water, which may irritate skin.

HOW TO WASH YOUR FACE: A STEP-BY-STEP GUIDE

What's the best way to wash your face? Some women swear by liquid cleansers, while others are faithful to traditional soap and water. The truth is, there is no one best way to wash your face. As usual, it depends upon factors such as your particular skin type and makeup routine. In general:

- Use a mild soap or cleanser suited to your skin type.
- Be sure to remove all traces of makeup.
- Wash your face gently. Never *scrub* your face.
- Rinse your face well with lukewarm—never hot—water.
- Pat—do not rub—your face dry with a soft towel.

Different Cleansers for Different Skin Types

Different skin types, of course, require different cleansers. The most inexpensive cleanser is highly underrated soap. Whereas in the past soap was extremely alkaline and could irritate delicate skin, many beauty soaps today have a low alkalinity and also contain valuable moisturizers. Superfatted moisturizing soaps are fine for women who have normal to dry skin. Creamy cleansers are also appropriate for normal to dry skin; they contain special emollients that moisturize and soften as they cleanse.

Women who have very dry or sensitive skin, on the other hand, are better off with gentle facial cleansers in place of soap and water. Light-textured products including lotions, milks, and mousses are all good alternatives for this skin type. Gentle cleansers remove dirt and makeup without irritating skin. Many are available without dyes or fragrances, ingredients that can irritate dry or sensitive skin.

Women with oily skin, large pores, or combination skin may choose cleansers that also contain toners to remove excess oil and tighten skin. Although there is no way to permanently eliminate enlarged pores, the ingredients in toners may make pores appear smaller for a short time. Some cleansers also exfoliate, or speed the shedding of dead skin cells. Try to avoid cleansers and other skin care products that are *too* drying to skin; there may be a rebound effect in which glands are stimulated to overproduce oil to compensate for once oily skin that has become overdry.

Sorting Out Soaps and Cleansers

- **Traditional soaps** are ordinary alkaline bars that are usually made through the milling process, in which soap chips are blended and compressed. These soaps are fine if you have normal skin, but their high alkaline or pH level may be irritating to women who have dry skin.
- **Detergent soaps** are sometimes considered harsher than traditional soaps, but manufacturers generally add moisturizers or emollients to them to soften their detergent effect. Detergent soaps also have the advantage of being nonalkaline, or pH-balanced.
- **Superfatted soaps** contain fatty materials such as cold cream, cocoa butter, neutral fats, and lanolin. Women who have dry skin may prefer to use superfatted soaps—but should not neglect to use a regular moisturizer afterward.
- **Castile soaps** are simply made with olive oil rather than other forms of fat.

- **Transparent soaps** contain more fat, like superfatted soaps, as well as glycerin. Unfortunately, transparent soaps do not lather well and are somewhat more costly than other soaps. Transparent soaps are best for women who have sensitive but oily skin.
- **Medicated soaps** may be prescribed by dermatologists for patients who have acne. It's not wise to wash with medicated or abrasive soaps unless your dermatologist specifically prescribes them, since overuse can result in dryness, redness, and irritation.
- **Deodorant soaps** contain antibacterial agents that can help diminish normal body odor, which is due to the action of bacteria on sweat secretions. Deodorant soaps must be used on a regular basis to be effective. It is not clear that most people really need these soaps, since a deodorant or antiperspirant must still be applied afterward. You should *not* use deodorant soap on your face.

Today's Woman Prefers Water to Oil

The majority of women today, no matter what their skin type, prefer oil-free cleansers and other skin care products. Oil—even healing oil such as vitamin E—can clog pores and lead to skin problems in many women, especially those with oily or acne-prone skin.

Water, on the other hand, makes for a youthful finish, and has become a major ingredient in many skin care products. Water hydrates, relaxes, and rejuvenates the skin, and a wide variety of spray-on water atomizers and rehydrating body mists are available today. After hydration skin is better able to absorb moisturizers.

To Bathe or to Shower? And How Often?

Americans are among the cleanest people in the world, most of us bathing or showering at least once a day. The rest of the world regards this habit with astonishment.

The truth is that it is not necessary for most people to undertake these ablutions on a daily basis. Unless you exercise and/or sweat excessively, or have very oily skin, daily cleansing of your complete body is unwarranted. Sponging those parts of your body that emit odor—the genital region, the armpits, and the feet—is sufficient.

Yet since most of us are pleasantly accustomed to our daily cleansing routines and are not disposed to abandon them, we should at least exercise caution by not allowing them to dry out our skin. Showering, for example, is far less drying to the skin than bathing.

If you have dry skin, it's best to shower and sponge-bathe. If you still love your baths, keep them down to one or two a week at most, limit your time spent in the bathtub, and avoid overly hot, drying water. Also, do not use regular soap. Bath oil can be somewhat helpful, but alone it is not a sufficient moisturizer; be sure to apply a whole body moisturizer after your bath. Those with sensitive skin should altogether avoid bath oils, gels, carbonated tablets, and bubble baths that contain fragrance, dye, and other potentially irritating ingredients.

MOISTURIZER

Most women experience dry skin as they age and can benefit from using a moisturizer. For best results, moisturizers should be applied to skin that is still damp from cleansing. When a moisturizer is applied to damp skin, the skin can hold more water, which temporarily plumps up fine, parched lines.

Classic moisturizers contain emollients that are appropriate for normal to dry skin. The major ingredient in these products is water, followed by emollients and an emulsifier to keep the water and emollients from separating. The most commonly used emollients are petrolatum, lanolin, and mineral oil.

Lighter lotions and gels are better suited for normal to oily skin. Women with this skin type should always begin with a small amount of moisturizer, and add to it as necessary. Too much moisturizer can give your face a shiny or greasy appearance, and may clog pores. In fact, the best moisturizers for all skin types are labelled as noncomedogenic.

Women who have very dry or sensitive skin should avoid moisturizers that contain fragrances and preservatives, which can irritate skin. Dry or aging skin can benefit most from the new high-tech moisturizers that contain concentrated emollients and alpha hydroxy acids.

Moisturize Your Whole Body

When we talk about moisturizing, we often are referring to the special moisturizing needs of your face. But as the years go by, keep in mind that your whole body is growing drier and craves moisture. The skin of your neck is as thin and fine as that of your face, and can experience insidious sun damage and dryness. Whenever you moisturize your face, add the same moisturizer—preferably one that also includes sun protection—to your neck as well.

Your hands and nails also require moisturizer to continue looking young and healthy. Using moisturizer that contains sunscreen can help prevent age spots from developing on your hands. Last but not least, do not neglect those areas of your body that are subjected to the most wear and tear: your feet and elbows. If you fail to properly moisturize feet and elbows, skin may thicken and grow rough, dry, and scaly due to constant friction and pressure.

WHEN TO SEE YOUR DERMATOLOGIST

Sometimes tightness and dry skin are the signs of more serious underlying skin problems. Flaking and dry, scaly patches on your face, for example, may be due to dermatitis. In this case, a heavy moisturizer may clog your pores and worsen the condition. If your regular moisturizer is no longer effective, it's best to see your dermatologist to diagnose and treat the problem.

SUNSCREEN

The American Academy of Dermatology recommends that everyone who spends time outdoors, no matter what time of year, use sunscreen on a daily basis. Remember that protecting your skin from the sun is the single most effective way to prevent skin damage that can lead to premature aging and skin cancer. Sun protection is necessary not only for summer days lounging on the beach or sailboat. You should apply sunscreen every time you go outdoors, whether it is commuting to and from work, out riding your bike, mowing the lawn, or raking leaves.

When choosing a sunscreen, again consider your skin type. In this case, are you fair-skinned or dark-skinned? Do you tan easily or do you tend to burn? Do you freckle easily? These are all important considerations. While everyone requires sun protection, fair-skinned people who burn easily are at the greatest risk of sun damage. And freckles, like age spots, are a sign of sun damage. You must also take into account factors such as how long you will be exposed to the sun; the strength of the sun; the relative sensitivity of your skin; and whether you require waterproof sun protection. Also, what time of year is it and how close are you to the equator? Are you hiking or skiing at high altitudes?

A broad spectrum sunscreen with an SPF of 15 or higher is

generally your best bet. Broad spectrum sunscreens protect your skin from harmful UVA as well as UVB rays. Sunscreen should be evenly applied at least fifteen minutes before exposure to the sun, to allow time for protective ingredients to interact with the skin. If you tend to have allergies, be certain to use a PABA-free product. (See Chapter 4 for a complete discussion of the impact that sun can have on your skin, and how to protect yourself from sun damage.)

ARE EXPENSIVE PRODUCTS BEST?

Prestigious, high-end cosmetics companies proudly extol the virtues of their new combination products that do it all. Yet companies that offer popularly priced drugstore brands have long been selling products such as cleansers that moisturize, moisturizers that provide sun protection, and even oil-free moisturizers. And, as you will see later in this chapter, you can also easily and economically make your own skin care products. The truth is, you don't have to spend a lot of money to take good care of your skin.

SIMPLE SKIN CARE PROGRAMS FOR EVERY SKIN TYPE

HOW TO CARE FOR NORMAL SKIN
- Wash your face on a daily basis with a low-alkaline soap or cleanser.
- Apply a light moisturizer.
- Protect yourself with a broad spectrum sunscreen with an SPF of at least 15 whenever you are exposed to the sun.
- Avoid products that are overly oily or drying.

HOW TO CARE FOR DRY SKIN

- Cleanse your skin with superfatted soaps or creamy cleansers. Avoid highly alkaline products.
- Moisturize your skin on a daily basis.
- If your skin is extremely dry, consider applying a heavier cream at night in addition to your daily moisturizer.
- Protect your skin from further dryness and photoaging by using a broad spectrum sunscreen with an SPF of at least 15 whenever you are exposed to the sun.
- If your skin is sensitive as well as dry, avoid products that contain potentially sensitizing ingredients, such as fragrances and dyes.

HOW TO CARE FOR OILY SKIN

- Wash your face with cleansers that also contain toner, which will help control oily skin.
- Avoid overly drying cleansers, which may create an undesirable rebound effect.
- Do not use medicated or abrasive soaps unless they are prescribed by your dermatologist.
- Follow cleansing with the application of a small amount of a noncomedogenic, oil-free moisturizer.
- Use gentle alcohol-free toners at least once or twice a week to remove excess oil.
- Avoid the temptation to overscrub or exfoliate oily or acne-prone skin; this may actually worsen your condition.
- Apply a noncomedogenic, oil-free broad spectrum sunscreen with an SPF of at least 15 whenever you are exposed to the sun.
- Use only noncomedogenic, oil-free cosmetics on your skin.
- In cases of prolonged or severe acne, see your dermatologist.

HOW TO CARE FOR COMBINATION SKIN

- Use a gentle cleanser to wash your face on a daily basis.
- Apply a light moisturizer to dry parts of your face (usually the sections that are not in the more oily T-zone—comprised of the chin, nose, and forehead).
- Use gentle alcohol-free toners at least once or twice a week to remove excess oil from the T-zone.
- Apply a noncomedogenic, oil-free broad spectrum sunscreen with an SPF of at least 15 whenever you are exposed to the sun.
- Use only noncomedogenic, oil-free cosmetics on your skin.

CHOOSING ADDITIONAL SKIN CARE PRODUCTS

Beyond the basic skin care products that we need every day are special treatments, such as exfoliators, masks, and toners. Products such as these can be used to customize your skin care routine—some can be applied on a daily basis, while others should be employed more sparingly.

EXFOLIATORS

Mild exfoliation is commonly advised by beauty experts. Behind the rough, dry, and abused outer layer of your skin, so the theory goes, is a soft layer of unspoiled translucent skin, smooth and fine as that of a baby. The trick is to remove the dead cells of the epidermis through the use of an exfoliator or scrub, thereby exposing this silky, polished layer. Exfoliators may be applied with washcloths or with more abrasive loofahs.

Yet dermatologists advise caution in the use of these "magic bullets." Although scrubs do indeed slough off dead skin cells, they may also leave skin dry, red, and irritated. Use them once or twice a week at most. To avoid damaging your skin with exfoliators, avoid scrubbing too hard and apply moisturizer after use. Exfoliators should not be used on acne or broken skin. Although they are not a long-term solution, exfoliators can effectively remove flaky skin.

MASKS

Masks can be used approximately once a week to individualize your regular skin care routine. Like a facial, a mask provides a psychological time-out, a rare moment of relaxation in the otherwise hectic lives of most women. Also like facials, the effects of a mask are temporary; they will not, for example, clear up acne or wrinkles.

There are two basic types of masks; those for dry skin and those for oily skin. For dry skin, there are moisturizing masks with bases of cream or oil. Masks with bases of clay or mud, on the other hand, are designed to remove surface sebum from oily skin and unclog pores. Astringent ingredients in masks designed for oily skin can also temporarily shrink enlarged pores.

All masks provide some degree of exfoliation, leaving your skin rosy and smooth. Carefully follow the package directions. As a general rule, masks should be left on no longer than five minutes, and must be removed gently to avoid facial irritation.

TONERS

Today's toners are kinder, gentler versions of yesterday's astringents. Toners (also known as clarifiers, refreshers, and purifiers) remove excess oil and tighten skin. Most dermatologists believe that a good cleanser does the job for normal skin, making toners appropriate primarily for those concerned with oily skin or large pores. While some women use a toner every day, sufficient application is probably once or twice a week.

Most toners are now low in alcohol or alcohol-free. This is in contrast to old-fashioned astringents, which had a high alcohol content that stripped skin of its natural moisturizers. Yet ingredients in some toners—such as alcohol, salicylic acid, and resorcinol—may still have a drying effect on skin. In addition, you would be wise to avoid toners that still include potential irritants such as camphor, menthol, and eucalyptus oil. Whatever toner, astringent, clarifier, or refresher you choose, be sure to apply an oil-free moisturizer afterward.

THE TRUTH ABOUT FACIALS

Facials offered at salons are relaxing moments in the busy lives of women and can offer a temporary cosmetic and psychological lift. Steam is often used in facials to open pores for deep cleaning. If you have dry skin, your facialist may massage heavy lotions into your skin. Depending on your skin type, facialists may also apply masks to hydrate skin or remove oil and tighten pores. The stimulation of a facial can bring blood vessels to the surface of the skin, giving your face a rosy glow.

The effects of facials, however, are temporary. Moreover, facials should be administered only by experienced and certified persons in very clean settings. Aggressive steaming, vacuuming pores, and the use of sharp instruments should all be avoided in facials. Steaming and steam machines are especially inappropriate if you have sensitive or acne-prone skin. And remember: only your dermatologist can treat serious skin problems.

CHOOSING THE RIGHT COSMETICS

The single most important fact you need to know about cosmetics is that they are very safe. Even though the cosmetic industry is not regulated by the FDA, there are laws to mandate that cosmetics are safe and minimally active on the skin.

Cosmetics are defined by the Federal Food, Drug, and Cosmetic (FD&C) Act as "beautifying" or "promoting attractiveness." This is to distinguish cosmetics from drugs, which are strictly regulated by the FDA since they have a direct effect on the function of the human body. There is an excellent voluntary safety panel that has reviewed a majority of the active ingredients and found them safe.

When choosing cosmetics, keep in mind that they will only have a superficial effect upon your skin. For the treatment of serious cases of acne or for the removal of wrinkles, for example, you must see your dermatologist. Below is a guide to choosing the right cosmetics.

CELEBRATE YOUR HERITAGE

A slew of new skin care lines have been specially formulated for women of color. While marketing forces obviously play a role in this trend, dark skin does indeed have special characteristics. Many moisturizers, for example, are too greasy for the skin of many black women, so new collections offer oil-free moisturizers.

Cosmetics for women of color are designed to highlight features such as rich skin tones, naturally curly hair, and almond eyes. Many products are alcohol-free, since alcohol is drying and can leave ashy overtones on dark skin. Comedogenic ingredients should especially be avoided by dark-skinned women, since acne on dark skin can lead to very visible scarring. Foundations for women of color are available in shades such as warm bronze, copper, and mahogany. Shades of lipstick include deep chocolate and ruby red.

FOUNDATION

While many women still begin the application of makeup with a light foundation, the pancake foundation of yesteryear is virtually extinct. What we used to call foundations are more commonly known today as finishes or liquid powders, and are evenly applied over the entire face and neck before any other makeup. Modern combinations of liquid and powder provide sheer and natural-looking coverage, simplify your beauty routine, and are often more economical as well. In response to women's concerns, most foundations are available in oil-free formulas, and many foundations also protect your skin with SPFs ranging from 8 to 15.

BLUSH

Blush can add color to faces, which is a definite plus now that we are aware of the serious hazards posed by exposure to the sun and tanning. If you have oily or acne-prone skin, choose gel or powder blushes instead of heavy creams. Also be sure to match your blush to your skin and hair color:

- Fair-skinned blondes may opt for peach or rose shades.
- Redheads often look best with honey blush.
- Brunettes and women of color may want to try deep shades of berry or plum.

CONCEALERS

Many women use concealers to cover blemishes or scars. Under-eye concealers can be applied around the whole eye to hide veins as well as circles under eyes. After application, concealers can be set with a soft, translucent powder. If you have oily or acne-prone skin, be sure to use an oil-free concealer.

EYE MAKEUP

The skin around your eyes and eyelids is among the most sensitive on your body, and extra consideration should be taken in choosing products for this area. Care should also be exercised in applying these products.

Mascara

Today's mascaras are formulated to plump up lashes, promote fullness, and avoid unsightly clumps. Brushes are designed to smooth away rough edges, and some brushes have a variety of textures to achieve different cosmetic effects. In concert with today's joint emphases on simplicity and choice, many mascaras available today are waterproof.

Eye Shadow

Modern eye shadows are made with softer and subtler colors. Designed to bring eyes to life, earth tones are emphasized, and harsh colors are generally not considered as satisfying. The best shadow combination for women is matte, a mixture of talc and pigment that is least likely to irritate eyes.

Eyeliner

Eyeliners are now available in the form of pencils, cakes, and tubes. If you use eyeliner, be careful not to pull at the delicate skin of your eye, and do *not* apply to inner lids since this may lead to irritation and infection.

Eye Creams

Eyes look best when the skin around them is firm and smooth. Eye creams are reputed to revitalize the skin around your eyes, temporarily adding moisture and reducing the appearance of puffiness and fine lines. But remember that eye creams are a cosmetic, not a drug; they cannot turn back the clock.

WASH OR REPLACE YOUR BRUSHES, PUFFS, AND SPONGES ON A REGULAR BASIS

Brushes, puffs, and sponges make blending makeup easy—but it's important to wash or replace these tools on a regular basis. Applicators may become breeding grounds for bacteria after as few as three or four uses. To protect your skin, don't borrow or share personal makeup items; you may end up borrowing or sharing a bacterial infection. Replace mascara brushes every three months. Wash powder puffs and foundation sponges weekly and replace them once a month.

FRAGRANCE

The basic dermatological concern for fragrances: Avoid those that cause allergic reactions. Test on a small patch of skin before surrounding yourself in a new scent.

LIPSTICK

Your lips require moisture and sun protection. Most new lipsticks are designed, therefore, to meet these requirements as well as to give your lips a cosmetic color boost. New lip colors are formulated to stay on your lips. They set in a minute or two, and cannot be kissed off. Modern reds come in every shade, from rich, creamy mattes, to soft, sheer stains. Ruby red and deep chocolate are popular shades for women of color, while trends such as vanilla-flavored lip gloss come and go.

LIP BALMS

Those of us who suffer from chronically chapped lips require more than ordinary lipstick. Rough, dry, and cracked lips are mainly a behavioral problem: In most cases, they are a result of licking your lips. But until you break the lip-licking habit, apply moisturizing lip balms on a regular basis. Lip balms are available as clear waxy sticks or ointments, and most contain valuable protective sunscreen. Use whenever your lips feel dry, especially in cold weather, if you have a cold, and when you go to bed at night. Many women use petroleum jelly as the traditional home remedy of choice for chapped lips—but since petroleum jelly does not contain sunscreen, use it only at night.

THE TRUTH ABOUT HYPOALLERGENIC PRODUCTS

If you have hypersensitive, reactive skin, it's best to use hypoallergenic products. However, since the tests used by cosmetic manufacturers are not regulated by any federal agency, consumers have no way of knowing the extent of the testing that has taken place.

Try to stick with longtime hypoallergenic cosmetic manufacturers who have a good track record responding to the special needs of those with sensitive skin. It's also a good idea to test all new skin care products on a small patch of skin. If you do not experience redness or irritation, you can gradually begin to use the product more freely. Keep in mind that fragrances and preservatives in cosmetics are especially likely to produce allergic reactions in susceptible women.

ALTERNATIVE SKIN CARE

More and more women today are choosing natural skin care products as an alternative to commercial cosmetics. Some women choose food from the kitchen shelf or refrigerator to make their own cosmetics at home. Many others purchase botanical products in local health food stores, and an increasing number of mainstream drugstores and department stores are beginning to carry these products as well. Because of their growing popularity, alternative skin care products are becoming more expensive. Keep in mind that because most natural products do not contain preservatives, they should be used soon after you make or purchase them. Limited testing has been done on these products and they may irritate sensitive skin. Following are some natural ways to address some special skin care concerns:

- Apply natural moisturizers to soften your skin. Natural moisturizers include aloe oil, apricot oil, avocado oil, cocoa butter, coconut oil, jojoba oil, olive oil, sesame oil, and shea butter.
- Use elder and aloe products to both moisturize your skin and whiten age spots.
- Make an herbal skin tonic of chamomile and lavender to revive dull and tired skin.
- Make your own facial steambath by adding a few drops of peppermint oil to a pot of hot water. Cover your head with a towel and rest your face over the pot to cleanse pores. Make sure the water is not too hot. (*Note:* Steaming is not recommended if you have sensitive skin, broken skin, or an active flare-up of acne.)
- Use products made from the herb lady's mantle to help shrink large pores.
- Use products made from sage, a good natural astringent, to tighten skin.
- Tone your skin with diluted witch hazel, a natural astringent.
- Make an exfoliating scrub from natural abrasive materials. These include ground cornmeal, oatmeal, apricot seeds, and almonds; simply combine them with a small amount of water or use a base of plain yogurt. (Reminder: Do not attempt to scrub or exfoliate if you have sensitive skin, broken skin, or an active flare-up of acne.)

TODAY'S GOAL: SIMPLE YET
EFFECTIVE SKIN CARE

The philosophy of simplifying your skin care routine makes sense in today's busy world. Yet since none of us are willing to sacrifice quality skin care, women today are devising streamlined programs for their particular skin types that are increasingly simple yet effective. In the next chapter, you will see that this same approach applies to hair and nail care.

CHAPTER 8

CARING FOR YOUR HAIR AND NAILS

Healthy skin is best complemented by healthy, well-groomed hair and nails. Like the top layer of the skin, hair and nails are composed primarily of the nonliving protein keratin—the same tough substance that makes up the horns of animals.

Today's philosophy of Less Is Better applies to hair and nails as well as skin. Like your skin, your hair and nails require moisture and conditioning to give them strength and enable them to withstand the daily wear and tear of friction, tension, and brushing.

In the proliferation of hair and nail care products, some may be very effective and others of questionable merit. In this chapter, we'll sort through the many products and procedures available, and help you choose the ones that are right for you.

YOUR HEALTHY HAIR

For prehistoric humans, hair was a necessity. Today women may consider hair to be alternately their crowning glory or the bane of their existence. The average head contains between 80,000 and 120,000 hair follicles, and the root of each hair is contained in the hair follicle in the epidermis. Each strand of your hair is composed of two primary layers: the *cuticle*, or outer layer, which protects the inner layer, or *cortex*, from splitting and fraying.

HOW YOUR HAIR GROWS

Hair normally grows and rests in scattered cycles, with some hairs in the growing phase of the cycle while others are being shed. Otherwise, like some animals, we would experience alternating periods of hairiness and baldness. Hairs on the scalp have growing cycles that range from two to six years, with hair growing at an average rate of a third to a half an inch each month, and most women normally lose fifty to one hundred hairs on a daily basis. In warm weather, blood circulation is enhanced, and the pace of hair growth increases by 10 to 15 percent. In cold weather and during illness, hair cells slow production. This is because circulation is more sluggish at these times, as blood is required to keep internal organs warm.

THE CYCLES OF HAIR GROWTH

Healthy hair grows and rests in cycles. The natural length of your growing cycle will determine whether your hair will be short or long. As women age, the rate of hair growth and hair volume declines.

Each cycle of hair growth contains three phases:

- The anagen is the growing phase.
- The telogen is the resting and falling-out phase.
- The catagen is the transitional phase.

ETHNICITY AND YOUR HAIR

The color, thickness, and curliness of your hair depends to some extent on your ethnic background and genetic predisposition. Blonds, for example, have about 120,000 scalp hairs, brunettes have some 100,000, and redheads about 80,000. Appearances, of course, can be deceiving. Since redheads have fewer but thicker scalp hairs, their hair may seem more abundant than the thin, fine hair that is typical of blonds.

How curly your hair is depends primarily on the shape of the cortex of your hair shafts:

- A cross section of the cortex of Asian hair is round, and Asian women have straight hair.
- A cross section of the cortex of black hair is flattened and curved, and black women have curly hair.
- A cross section of the cortex of white women's hair is slender, cylindrical, and varies in curve, with the degree of its curve determining the amount of curve in hair, from straight to curly.

THE STAGES AND AGES OF YOUR HAIR

Your hair passes through a multitude of stages as you age. There is a great deal of overlapping, and every woman's hair is unique. Still, there are certain sets of characteristics generally shared by each decade—from the thick and glossy hair of youth, to more-difficult-to-manage thin and graying hair as we age.

As with skin, there are many products available to cope with changing hair as we age. For example, new shampoos and conditioners are available to cover gray, and moisturizers and volumizers can minimize the impact of thinning hair. In this section, we'll trace hair through the decades, and explore some of the natural and cosmetic ways to cope with the many changes that take place over time.

Your Youthful Hair

In your youth, you have an opportunity to establish the good hair care habits you'll need for a lifetime. Many women's hair is thickest at the age of twenty, and normal hair requires a minimum of care during these years. In many young adults, on the other hand, excess facial and scalp oil build up to clog pores and cause acne. If you have oily or acne-prone skin, it's important to wash your hair on a daily basis to control oily scalp conditions (such as seborrheic dermatitis) that can exacerbate acne.

Healthy hair, like healthy skin, is also a reflection of a healthy lifestyle. Dry and brittle hair, for example, may be the result of an eating disorder, overexposure to the sun, or mistreating your hair through excessive bleaching, perming, or brushing. Good hair care during the twenties is comprised of regular washing, grooming, conditioning as necessary, and avoiding repeated chemical treatments such as dyes and perms.

In Your Thirties

As you enter your thirties, you're probably beginning to notice—and pluck out—the first strands of gray hair. Hair turns gray because we tend to produce less pigment as we grow older. Your hair is also a little finer in your thirties, and it will continue to thin as you grow older.

Yet there's no reason that thirtysomething hair cannot remain healthy and shiny as long as you are willing to expend a little extra effort. Limit your use of hot curlers and, if you must use a blow dryer, keep it on a low setting. Good grooming is also more important now, so frequent trims will help. Regular conditioning is also a must.

In Your Forties

If you're like many women, the gray hairs are probably coming in too thickly now for plucking to be of much use. You may want to try a semipermanent or temporary hair coloring to camouflage your gray. This can help you decide on whether you want to embark on a longer-lasting and more permanent hair-coloring routine, or continue to cover gray with temporary coloring, or simply go gray. Many women feel that when gray hair is cut well and properly moisturized to remain shiny it can be as attractive as any other hair color.

Your hair will also grow considerably thinner, drier and duller as you progress through your forties. But there are steps you can take to counteract this natural process. Shampoos that add moisture, thickness, and volume to your hair are helpful. And now's the time to invest in those weekly leave-in conditioning treatments (although some women find that olive oil works just as well!). Good grooming is even more important, as regular trims lessen the necessity for extended styling sessions with the damaging heat of a blow dryer.

In Your Fifties and Beyond

Hair, like skin and nails, is controlled to some extent by hormonal production. Consequently, after menopause women's hair patterns often change dramatically. Yet if you continue to eat properly, exercise, and pay attention to the changing needs of your hair, it can remain healthy and attractive.

Although we usually think of men as having the problem of thinning hair, women experience it as well. Estrogen stimulates hair growth, and the absence or reduction of estrogen after menopause—coupled with the greater presence of male hormones called androgens—contributes to hair loss in women. To prevent the look of excessive hair loss, try using shampoos that add volume to hair.

You may also consider a short, layered cut to add volume and de-emphasize thinning hair. (Long hair is no longer as flattering as we grow older.) And remember to cover your thin and graying hair when you are exposed to sunlight; because hair is thinner, your scalp is more likely to burn, while gray hair can take on a yellowish tint when exposed to sun, salt, and chlorine. Scarves, broad-brimmed hats, and bathing caps are helpful accessories.

CARING FOR YOUR HAIR

People in general use too many products on their hair. You yourself probably own many hair-management products—but do they give you the look you want? The starting point to effective hair care and styling is to determine what type of hair you have. Then you can choose a simple routine to get the look you're after.

Hair type is defined according to texture and condition. Textures range from fine to medium to coarse, and conditions may be oily, normal, or dry. Many hair care products are labeled according to these categories, and this can be a great aid in determining the formula that will work best for you.

DETERMINING YOUR HAIR TYPE

TEXTURE	CHARACTERISTICS	PRODUCTS
Fine	Limp and flat; does not hold curl or style easily	Light products, such as mousse, that increase volume
Normal or Medium	Easily maintains curl or style	Your choice
Coarse	Coarse or curly hair is easier to comb when wet; hard to manage; may be frizzy	Heavy creams and gels that decrease volume

CONDITION		
Oily	Requires daily washing	Oil-free, fast-drying products
Normal	Requires washing after two days; shiny	Your choice
Dry	Dull; frizzy; staticky	Products rich in oil; conditioners

SHAMPOOS

The key to healthy hair is maintaining a proper moisture balance. Today's shampoo formulas can add health, vitality, and shine to your hair with no oils or heaviness.

Shampoos ordinarily combine two basic ingredients—detergent and water—and come in three formulations: for normal, dry, and oily hair. There are also shampoos specially formulated for chemically treated hair, shampoos that add body and volume to your hair, moisturizing shampoos, and dandruff shampoos. It's important to choose the formula that is best suited to your own hair type. You may opt for one of the specially formulated shampoos:

- Shampoos for chemically treated hair have a low pH to compensate for the higher pH of treated hair, are low in alkaline, and include a light conditioner.
- Shampoos that add volume to hair are made from protein formulas that protect the delicate balance of your hair while coating it to add thickness and body.
- Moisturizing shampoos contain conditioning ingredients—such as sugars, botanicals, or natural plant oils—that add moisture back into dry, brittle hair.
- Dandruff shampoos contain ingredients such as coal tar to control flaking of the scalp.

MIXING UP YOUR SHAMPOOS

It's a good idea to keep several different types of shampoo in your bathroom and switch back and forth among them. If you have been using a regular cleansing shampoo over the last week, for example, you may want to use a moisturizing shampoo to soothe dry hair. A cleansing shampoo, on the other hand, can wash away product buildup if you ordinarily wash your hair with a moisturizing shampoo.

CONDITIONERS

Yesterday's cream rinses are today's conditioners, and they are available for two main purposes:

- **Body-building** conditioners are designed to add bounce to your hair. They are generally oil-free and rich in proteins that coat the shafts of your hair.
- **Moisturizing** conditioners are appropriate for dry and brittle hair and can be especially helpful for chemically treated hair.

There are also two categories of conditioners:

- **Daily** conditioners are designed to be washed off easily after every shampoo.
- **Deep** conditioners—and leave-in conditioners—have ingredients that can penetrate hair shafts when you leave them on for the designated five to twenty minutes. Leave-in conditioners are especially helpful for coarse hair.

BLOW-DRYING AND BRUSHING YOUR HAIR

Beehive dryers are obsolete, and blow-drying has come a long way. Some dryers have attached combs or diffusers that can add body to fine hair. Setting the dryer on a cooler setting minimizes damage to hair and can help your hair hold curl.

There are also some new thoughts about brushing out your hair. No longer are one hundred strokes a night recommended. Today's philosophy of Less Is Better also applies to brushing your hair. Choose a brush with natural, round-ended bristles, and gently brush your hair. When detangling hair, use a wide-toothed comb to avoid breaking strands and creating split ends.

HAIR CARE TIPS

- Avoid very hot showers, which may dry your scalp and increase your risk of dandruff.
- Choose a shampoo appropriate to your type of hair. Newly color-treated hair, for example, requires an extra gentle formula so that it will not affect your new color.
- Wash your hair just once each time; no need to "repeat."
- Try adding one ounce of vinegar to shampoo each week to wash out residue from hair spray, gel, etc.
- When grooming wet or damp hair, use a wide-toothed comb instead of a brush.
- When blow-drying your hair, never use the highest heat setting.
- Use a diffuser when you blow-dry permed hair.
- Style your hair on lower speeds—it's actually more effective.
- Keep your brush and comb clean. Regularly remove hair from them, and soak them in warm water once a week.
- Do not share your brush or comb with anyone.
- Avoid overuse of heated styling tools such as curling irons and rollers.
- Don't pull your hair back in very tight ponytails; never use plain rubber bands.

CHOOSING THE RIGHT STYLING PRODUCTS

Sprays, spritzes, mousses, and gels are among the many styling products available today, and they have one thing in common: They are all designed to hold your style in place. They do this through the use of polymers, a base of large molecules. Products that promise a firm hold usually contain alcohol; lighter styling products, for softer styles, are water-soluble and alcohol-free.

Here are some of the more popular styling products available today:

- **Mousse**—which is sometimes called foam—coats and lifts strands of hair, adding body to fine or normal hair. Mousse is gentle and water-based and should be evenly combed through towel-dried hair.

- **Volumizers,** which can take forms ranging from lotions to sprays, add thickness and texture to hair. Made from a combination of proteins, resins, and silicones, volumizers coat fine-to-medium hair and make it heavier. Apply to damp hair and blow-dry.

- **Sculpting lotion**—or glaze or gloss—forms a light film on fine-to-medium hair, creating a light, dry hold. Comb into wet hair for a sleek look, or blow-dry for a softer look.

- **Spray gel**—or spritz gel or gel mist—can be used on fine hair for loose shaping. Spray on damp hair and style with fingers while blow drying.

- **Liquid gel**—sometimes known as sculpting gel—is best for medium to coarse hair. Gel, which should be applied to wet hair, dries hard for a wet, smooth look. Blow-dry and brush out if you want a softer effect.

- **Balm**—also known as cream or groom—contains moisturizers that protect your hair from heat styling. Best for medium to coarse dry hair, it can be combed into wet hair for a sleek look.

- **Polishing spray,** or spray sheen, adds moisture and shine and defrizzes medium to coarse dry hair. Polishing spray is made from botanicals and oils. Spray on dry, styled hair.

- **Silicone serum** uses a concentrated version of silicone to add shine and reduce the frizz of coarse, dry hair. Apply to wet or dry hair.

- **Silicone spray** adds shine to all hair types. Spray this combination of silicone and conditioners onto hair after you finish using other styling products.

- **Setting spray**—or lotion or gel—can be used on all hair types to give curls a firmer hold. Spray on both before and after curlers or rollers are set in place. Set-

ting spray coats hair strands with resins and conditioners, boosting the effects of rollers and curling
irons.

HOW TO GROW OUT BANGS

If you've ever tried it, you know that growing out bangs is a long and
frustrating process. For many women, it can take as much as two years for
bangs to grow out to an equal length with chin-length hair. Some women
simply give up and reach for the scissors. But a good technique to use
when growing out bangs is the application of gel or sculpting lotion to
bangs. Then simply brush them back off your face with the rest of your
hair. Adding a stylish headband can help keep stray strands tucked in.

CHEMICAL HAIR TREATMENTS

Chemical hair treatments, such as colors and perms, can
help you change and enhance the hair that biology has given
you. Yet even though today's chemical treatments are less harsh
than those employed in the past, too-frequent use can lead to
dull, dry hair or even hair loss. Any chemical applied to hair will
weaken the structure; fine hair is more vulnerable to damage
than thick, coarse hair. As always, Less Is Better. Try to add
variety to your hair care routine, interspersing your use of harsh
chemicals with gentler formulas. Also keep in mind that conditioners can at least temporarily strengthen treated or damaged
hair.

Changing Your Hair Color

One out of three American women colors her hair. Fortunately, the technology of hair color has made great strides, ren-
dering obsolete hair horror stories of black shoe polish jobs and
harsh peroxide blonds. Hair coloring techniques available range

from gentle temporary techniques to powerful ammonia-based permanent dyes.

Highlights with staying power are among the most popular hair coloring products today. Many companies make products called hair brighteners, which are designed to revitalize highlights between visits to the hairdresser. Another modern advantage is that when you want to go back to your natural color, you no longer have to simply let hair grow out. For women who want to change from dark hair to their own original lighter color, there are dye removers. There is also an option known as a "tintback," in which some of your colored hair is returned to its natural shade, resulting in a pleasant streaked effect.

The Five Major Types of Hair Coloring

- **Temporary hair color** is safe and gentle. Hair shafts are temporarily coated with darker shades or streaks of color that wash out easily. Temporary colors color the cuticle but do not penetrate the cortex, and cannot lighten hair.
- **Semipermanent hair color** falls squarely in between temporary and permanent hair coloring. These dyes penetrate the hair cuticle and cortex. Often available in shampoo-in form, semipermanent hair color lasts through approximately six cleansing shampoos.
- **Permanent hair color** is the only type that deeply penetrates the cortex and can lighten as well as darken hair. Most women who color their hair use this method. Color change takes place due to oxidation, and a powerful alkaline base, such as ammonia, is often used. If you are prone to allergic reactions, use a small test patch on your scalp twenty-four hours before applying permanent hair color.
- **Progressive hair color** products use metallic dye on the cuticle of the hair. Chemicals react with air to

form brown shades in the process of oxidation. Progressive hair colors cannot lighten hair.

- **Vegetable dyes** such as henna were formerly used primarily in Europe, but are becoming increasingly popular in the United States. These dyes are an especially good option for women who are allergic to chemicals in commercial dyes. The application of vegetable dyes is safe but often time-consuming, and henna cannot make dark hair lighter.

Opting for a Perm

Hair is made of protein molecules joined by chemical bonds. The texture of your hair—whether it is fine or coarse—and the shape of your hair—whether it is straight, curly, or somewhere in between—is determined by the particular configuration of protein molecules in your hair.

When you perm your hair, you break down this molecular structure and replace it with a new one. In the past, perms involved the use of harsh chemicals that often damaged hair. Today there are more options, as women with naturally curly hair seek to have it straightened, and women with straight hair apply chemicals to add bounce and curl.

After Chemical Treatments: Coping with Damaged Hair

A perm, by definition, permanently breaks down and rearranges the internal structure of your hair. It is rare that chemical products such as perms and dyes damage hair forever. However, a light perm ruffles the cuticle, while heavy damage indicates that you have disrupted the cortex of the hair. Repeated use of the chemicals in hair dyes and perms can result in dry and brittle hair.

It's important to take into account the fragility of chemically treated hair. Damaged hair is more porous, so everything it comes into contact with will penetrate it more deeply. This includes further exposure to chemicals (such as chlorine), sunlight, heat, the friction of brushing, and the tension of cornrows, braiding, or hairpieces. Try to reduce these potential causes of damage.

Undoing the harm that chemicals inflict upon hair is often a long-term project. On the positive side, the porous nature of damaged hair allows it more effectively to absorb strengthening conditions. Cut off split and broken ends as they grow out, and regularly apply conditioners to fortify damaged hair. If you are growing out a perm, blow-dry hair on a cool setting to blend the line where permed hair meets flat hair growing in.

PREGNANCY, NURSING, AND CHEMICAL HAIR TREATMENTS

Pregnancy and nursing can affect hair and therefore the effectiveness of chemical hair treatments. But even more important, it is possible—although it has not been proven—that chemicals in hair dye or perming products may affect a developing fetus. Women are usually advised to play it safe and put off hair perming or coloring until after giving birth and nursing.

CONTROLLING SCALP PROBLEMS

Sometimes the difficulties we experience with our hair are due to skin conditions of our scalp. Most problems are easily controlled with special over-the-counter dandruff shampoos. Other times, it may be necessary to pay a visit to your dermatologist.

DANDRUFF

Dandruff is actually a normal condition in which dead skin cells are sloughed off from the scalp. A condition known as pseudo-dandruff is created through the overuse of products such as gels, setting lotions, and sprays. For most people, regular hair washing keeps the shedding under control. Excessive dandruff, on the other hand, while not a serious condition can be quite embarrassing. An especially flaky scalp is usually associated with dry skin, and in many women it is more common in times of stress or illness, as well as in cold winter months. An over-the-counter dandruff shampoo may solve your problem.

SEBORRHEIC DERMATITIS

When the normal flaking of dandruff is accompanied by redness, scaling, and crusting of the scalp, you may be suffering from seborrheic dermatitis. Regular use of a dandruff shampoo—one that contains ingredients such as coal tar, zinc, or selenium—can often reduce cell turnover and keep this condition in check. If problems persist, however, see your dermatologist.

USING A DANDRUFF SHAMPOO

Dandruff shampoos should be used only when you definitely need them. In the recent past, these stronger shampoos were extremely drying to both the hair and the scalp—but today they also contain valuable moisturizers. Still, if you do find that you require a dandruff shampoo, use only a small amount and be sure to massage a moisturizer into your scalp after use.

THINNING HAIR: HOW TO CUT YOUR LOSSES

Most women have a particularly queasy and uncomfortable feeling about hair loss, or alopecia. For better or worse, our hair is an important part of the way we feel about ourselves and present ourselves to the world. Yet hair thinning and loss is one of a multitude of troubles experienced by many of us, female as well as male, as we grow older. A gradual thinning of hair naturally occurs with age, when new hair growth slows and each hair becomes thinner in diameter. Fortunately, while there are no miracle cures to report, there are a number of options you can explore to help you cope with this problem.

ONE IN FIVE

If you're a woman dealing with problems such as thinning hair or a widening of your natural part, you're not alone. About one out of every five women copes with this condition every day.

ANDROGENETIC ALOPECIA: THE MOST COMMON FORM OF HAIR LOSS

Androgenetic alopecia (AGA) is the most common form of baldness in both women and men and is caused by a combination of genetic predisposition and an excess of male hormones known as androgens. In women, this condition may begin anytime after puberty and is aggravated after menopause when our estrogen supply is severely depleted.

Androgenetic alopecia, or male pattern baldness, usually takes the form of a gradual decrease in the density of hair, especially across the top of women's heads. Women rarely go completely bald—but hair does become finer in texture. Hair loss in women is usually more moderate and much less noticeable than in men, in whom hair loss often involves balding at the crown and receding of the hairline.

The diagnosis of androgenetic alopecia is made on the basis of family history and the pattern of alopecia. There is no one highly effective therapy to halt the progression of AGA. Anti-seborrheal shampoos are recommended. Topically applied prescription minoxidil (Rogaine) may be helpful in partially restoring hair loss or reducing the rate of hair loss in some individuals. Antiandrogens may be prescribed to treating AGA in women, and hair transplantation is an option for both sexes.

ALOPECIA AREATA: AN AUTOIMMUNE DISORDER

Alopecia areata is a loss of hair in round or oval areas, which is not accompanied by scalp or skin inflammation. *Alopecia totalis* is a loss of all scalp hair and eyebrows, and *alopecia universalis* is a complete loss of body hair.

Alopecia areata and associated types of hair loss are autoimmune disorders, in which the body identifies its own hair follicles as foreign substances, inhibiting their growth and at times even destroying them altogether. People who have alopecia areata are often allergic individuals who suffer from other autoimmune disorders, such as atopic dermatitis, eczema, hay fever, thyroid disease, or vitiligo.

Young adults under the age of twenty-five are the group most frequently afflicted with this disease, and emotional problems are a common trigger of an alopecia attack. When alopecia areata occurs after puberty, 80 percent of those affected regrow hair. Alopecia universalis is fortunately rare, but recurrences of alopecia are a frequent problem.

There are various treatments for alopecia areata. Antisebhorreals, topical steroids, and occasionally systemic steroids may be helpful. The administration of PUVA (psoralens followed by careful exposure to UVA light) is often prescribed. Immune modulation is another mode of treatment. Women who experience alopecia areata usually find wigs helpful.

OTHER TYPES OF HAIR LOSS

Alopecia has a variety of causes, in addition to an excess of androgens or autoimmune problems. Other conditions that may lead to alopecia include seborrheic dermatitis, psoriasis, infections, and conditions of physical or chemical origin. Constant tension on the scalp from braiding, cornrows, or hairpieces can cause alopecia. Women should generally exercise restraint in the use of chemical treatments on their hair, since overuse can eventually lead to hair loss and baldness.

COPING WITH UNWANTED HAIR

On the other side of the coin are women who must cope with too much hair or hair in undesirable locations of the body. After menopause, changing hormonal levels in women often lead to hair growth on the face. But as women know, you don't have to wait until after menopause to deal with unwanted hair. Unlike other parts of the world, such as Europe, in American society it is considered unacceptable for women to have hair on our legs and underarms, let alone stray hairs escaping from the bottom of a bathing suit. Fortunately, there are many ways to remove undesirable hair.

HIRSUTISM: ANOTHER ANDROGEN-DEPENDENT DISORDER

Hirsutism, or excessive hair growth in male distribution, like alopecia has been linked to excess androgens. Elevated levels of androgens appear to disrupt normal hair growth patterns in two distinct ways: by hair loss that can lead to baldness (alopecia) or through immoderate and inappropriate hair growth (hirsutism). While genetic androgen disorders can occur at any time after the onset of puberty, hirsutism can be an especially difficult problem after menopause, when estrogen is lost and androgens become more dominant in women.

Prescription treatments for hirsutism include topical steroids, estrogen, and antiandrogens. Long-term anti-androgen therapy may be necessary. Many women also remove unwanted hair through plucking, shaving, waxing, and depilatories. The sudden onset of severe hirsutism suggests a tumor; a dermatologist or endocrinologist should be seen as soon as possible.

ELIMINATING UNWANTED HAIR: YOUR LEGS, UNDERARMS, AND BIKINI AREA

Following are methods women often use to remove excess hair from these areas:

- **Shaving** Shaving is by far the most common way in which women deal with hairy underarms and legs. Shaving is relatively fast, efficient, and inexpensive. It's always best to shave with the hair, not against it; otherwise, you may bury debris in skin and cause infection.

  Observe cleanliness throughout the process: Make sure that both the area to be shaved and the razor are clean. Many women prefer to use disposable razors for both sanitary reasons and convenience. If you use an electric shaver, skin should be dry; if you use a blade, it should be wet with water or foam. Shave in the direction of hair growth to avoid folliculitis. Directly after shaving, always apply moisturizer and never use irritating deodorants or antiperspirants.

- **Chemical Depilatories** Chemical depilatories break down the chemical structure of hair, so that hairs break and can be wiped off. The chief disadvantage to chemical depilatories is that they may cause irritation. Yet depilatories are very useful if you have warts or other skin problems that prevent you from shaving. If depilatories are irritating to skin, the application of over-the-counter topical steroids before or after use may be helpful.

- **Waxing** Waxing plucks hairs from beneath the skin's surface, so its effect is more lasting than that of shaving or chemical depilatories. Waxing, on the other hand, can be painful and irritating to the skin, so it should be done only by an experienced professional. The application of over-the-counter topical steroids shortly before or after waxing may counter irritation.

REMOVING FACIAL HAIR

In addition to shaving, women may try the following methods to remove or camouflage facial hair:

- **Bleaching** Bleaching is the simplest and least expensive way to cope with unwanted facial hair. It is also painless. The disadvantage of bleaching is that the hair, although less visible, is still present; occasionally, there are also problems with skin irritation.

- **Electrolysis** Electrolysis is the only permanent method of hair removal. In electrolysis, the root of the hair is destroyed with an electric current. Women who have hair on the upper lip or chin may want to investigate electrolysis. Yet the process is slow and expensive. Hair may grow back, and permanent scarring may occur if the procedure is not done correctly.

- **Tweezing** Some women regularly pluck their eyebrows with tweezers to make them finer and less bushy. Plucking out stray hairs with tweezers may be painful, but many women prefer it to the other alternatives. Plucked hairs usually grow back two to twelve weeks later.

WHAT'S NEW IN NAIL CARE

Your nails protect your fingertips and toes from injury and increase manual dexterity. Americans spend about 200 million dollars on nail care products each year, prompting cosmetic companies to flood the marketplace with an ever increasing number of products for your perusal. In order to remain both healthy and attractive, the nails on your hands and feet require proper care.

ABOUT YOUR NAILS

Fingernails and toenails are composed primarily of keratin, the same substance that is in your skin and hair. Nails grow an average of an eighth to a quarter of an inch each month. Fingernails may take six months to grow from base to tip, while toenails may take twice that long.

Nails have five parts:

- The *nail plate* is the medical term for the actual nail.
- The *nail bed* under the nail plate represents skin with blood vessels that nourish the nail.

- The *cuticle* is the fold of skin at the edges of your nail plate, which prevents dirt and bacteria from entering the nail.
- The *matrix,* located directly under the proximal cuticle, is the center where nail plate cells are regenerated.
- The *lunula* is the visible part of the matrix called half moon.

EFFECTIVE NAIL CARE

The most effective nail care consists of keeping your nails trimmed, clean, and dry. Yet many women extend their attention to nails far beyond these simple basics. Bad manicures are to blame for many nail problems. In an effort to make nails more attractive, for example, we often overcut cuticles and overuse nail products. Nails should also be allowed to go bare for a few days each month in order to let air reach them.

Many nail products today are made with gentler chemical formulas than in the past. Another advantages to modern polish is its chip-resistant formula. Nail polishes or enamels are fine for most women, although some become sensitized to chemicals in them and experience allergic reactions. If your skin tends to be easily irritated, nails may also split and scale. Look for fragrance-free and formaldehyde-free formulations of polishes and polish removers. Since polish removers contain ingredients such as acetone, which can be drying and irritating, choose removers that are nonacetone or contain lubricants. Rinse well after use.

HOW TO STRENGTHEN YOUR NAILS

As you grow older, keeping your nails well moisturized is the best way to keep them strong and healthy. It's important to use a moisturizer on a daily basis. Gelatin and calcium supplements, which are sometimes recommended to strengthen nails, have no proven value. Using a nail hardener may give your nails the temporary appearance of strength by preventing peeling and chipping—yet chemicals in nail hardeners may eventually backfire by resulting in irritation, discoloration and splitting of your nails. Steer clear of any nail hardeners that contain form-aldehyde. As usual, simple nail care is the most effective nail care.

FINGERNAILS AND HORSES' HOOVES

It's straight from the horse's mouth: Strengthening and moisturizing nail creams are being borrowed from the equestrian community. This new marketing ploy makes use of the heavy emollients in products for horses' hooves. It all started when grooms began to notice that after applying cream to strengthen horses' hooves, their own nails were becoming stronger. In fact, human nails are made from the same essential protein as horses' hooves. Collagen and vitamin E in hoof moisturizing formulas also penetrate human nails, strengthening, and protecting nails from breaks and splits. Horse shampoos have likewise gained in popularity among the human population, as horse shampoos seem to be restorative for two-legged as well as four-legged creatures.

ARTIFICIAL NAILS

It's often said that a manicurist can help you overcome bit-ten, broken, or damaged nails by gluing acrylic tips onto your own nails. The theory is that these artificial nails are left on until your nails grow to the point where you are comfortable remov-ing them. Yet we do not recommend this process. Nails grow slowly, and it takes about five months for a new nail to grow from the cuticle to the fingertip. In the meantime, acrylics can trap moisture under nails, leading to fungal and bacterial infec-tions, and possible allergic reactions.

NAIL CARE TIPS

- Less is better in nail care. Do not overmanicure your nails or apply nail products too frequently.
- Keep nails and hands well moisturized.
- Do not cut cuticles when manicuring your nails; moisturize and gently push them back.
- Use emery boards rather than metal nail files. The best files are the finest in texture and the least abusive to your nails.
- File your nails in one direction only.
- Don't bite your nails. Choose more productive—and less destructive— ways to handle your stress.
- Use protective gloves to wash dishes.

COMMON NAIL PROBLEMS

Most nail disorders are not serious. A trauma resulting in a broken nail, for example, usually simply disappears as your nail grows out over a six-month period. Yet some symptoms may be cosmetically disturbing, and others are a sign of a more serious underlying disease. In fact, doctors often examine fingernails as a clue to overall health. Following are some of the most common nail problems.

Brittle Nails

Brittle nails are the equivalent of dry skin, and if you suffer from dry skin you probably also have brittle nails. Brittleness can lead to painful horizontal or even vertical breaks in your nails.

A natural remedy to brittle nails is soaking them in warm water and applying a rich cream. Just as moisturizers temporarily plump up damp skin, your nails can be strengthened through the absorption of water and moisture. Also try to avoid contact with drying and irritating household detergents, which remove moisture and increase fragility of nails.

Fungal and Bacterial Infections

Both fingernails and toenails can be infected with fungi or bacteria. Fungi can grow on the hands and feet of people who are constantly exposed to wet or damp environments, and bacteria enter through broken nails and skin.

Your dermatologist can prescribe topical and oral antifungal medications or oral antibiotics to clear up infections. In the meantime, try to keep hands and feet dry; use talc, change socks frequently, avoid wearing shoes that are too tight, wear protective gloves when doing housework.

Hangnails

Hangnails are splits of the skin in the area surrounding the nail. Excessive dryness, vigorous clipping of the cuticle (over-manicuring), paper cuts, trauma to the skin, and nervous habits such as picking at or biting your nails often result in painful hangnails.

To prevent hangnails, keep your hands and nails well-moisturized at all times. Wear rubber gloves when you wash dishes or use harsh chemicals in cleaning. To treat hangnails, do *not* simply tear the hangnail off; this may only cause further pain and injury. Instead, carefully snip off the tip of dry skin with a fine set of scissors and moisturize with water and a moisturizing product.

Ingrown Toenails

Painful ingrown toenails are most common in the big toes and are often the result of wearing shoes that do not fit, picking at the toes, and overclipping the nails. Toenails should not be clipped too short or clipped in at sides. Left untreated, ingrown toenails may become infected, leading to tenderness, swelling, and a pussy discharge.

The best way to avoid ingrown toenails is to keep nails trimmed straight across (*not* curved or pointed) and wear shoes that fit properly (*not* pointy high heels that pinch toes). See your doctor for treatment, which may require soaking your feet in epsom salts, taking prescription oral antibiotics, and having minor surgery.

Nail Discolorations

Nail discolorations may be the result of a variety of causes, such as overapplication of nail polishes or hardeners, injury to the nail, contact with various chemicals or drugs, or the presence of an underlying disease. If discoloration persists, consult your dermatologist to help determine and treat its cause.

Nail Ridges

Lengthwise ridges on your nails, like wrinkles, are a sign of aging. Ridges may be due to overmanicuring or injury to the nail. At times they are a result of an underlying diseases, including arthritis of the hands, carpal tunnel syndrome, pneumonia, and psoriasis. Prominent ridges should be examined by your dermatologist.

HEALTHY HAIR AND NAILS: THE PERFECT COMPLEMENT TO HEALTHY SKIN

In these chapters we have seen that healthy hair, nails, and skin are the result of simple yet effective grooming routines. Much of what you have read here reflects our philosophy that

Less Is Better. If you don't overbrush or apply too many chemicals to your hair, if you moisturize your nails sufficiently yet resist the temptation to overmanicure them, and if you avoid overscrubbing your skin and protect yourself from sun exposure, you are well on your way to health.

CHAPTER 9

From a new recognition that sunbathing is the medical equivalent of cigarette smoking, to the use of products such as alpha hydroxy acids and Retin-A to counteract the effects of aging, to the kinder and gentler products to care for your skin, hair, and nails and simplify your health and beauty routines, it is clear that there are many advances taking place in the world of dermatology today. Whereas many of these are valid medical advances, other trends are really only passing fads. In this chapter we'll look more closely at what is new in skin care.

MELANOMA AND A FAULTY GENE

Recent studies have provided evidence of "markers" within an individual's genetic makeup that are related to the risk of developing melanoma, according to the National Center for Human Genome Research (part of the National Institutes of Health) and Myriad Genetics Inc. of Salt Lake City, Utah. About 10 percent of melanomas, the deadliest skin cancers, occur in people with an inherited tendency, and more evidence is accumulating that defects in a gene known as P-16 may be responsible in some part for the inherited tendency to melanoma. Defects in the gene may also play a role in noninherited melanoma.

In its normal state, the P-16 gene helps regulate cell division and prevents cancer. But a defective version of the gene apparently causes people to lose part of that protection, making them more vulnerable to melanoma. Two types of defects appeared in the P-16 gene in both studies, and researchers speculate that a second, unknown susceptibility gene may also play a role in this deadly disease. These and future findings may help in identifying people at high risk of melanoma, who should be observed more closely for early warning signs of the disease.

ULTRASOUND IN MELANOMA SURGERY

Identification of people who are susceptible to melanoma has not been the only recent advance in this area. The use of new high-frequency ultrasound imaging may prove extremely useful in defining the surgical treatment of melanoma, according to researchers at the University of Toronto Faculty of Medicine. Previous attempts to use ultrasound to gauge the depth of melanomas were inaccurate, probably due to overestimation of the depths of melanomas at the lower frequencies at which ultrasounds were conducted.

The success of ultrasound in judging melanomas is indeed good news to women who suffer from this extremely serious skin cancer. Moreover, ultrasound is considered so safe that it is even used to detect the health of developing fetuses in pregnant women. Ultrasound, therefore, both safe and noninvasive, may come to replace biopsies in presurgical planning.

A PROLIFERATION OF ANTIAGING PRODUCTS

With monikers ranging from reactivating to revitalizing to refreshing to replenishing, not to mention age-defying and turn-around, today's cosmetics emphasize that they are opening up a fountain of youth. Some are designed to be applied nightly, to work as you sleep. Others are to be used on a daily basis, protecting us from free radicals triggered by UV light, smoke, and pollution in the environment.

Cosmetic companies today are touting seaweed and other minerals from the sea to help protect and promote healthy skin. Other products are packed with antioxidants, enriched with supervitamins A, C, and E to fight free-radical damage. Vitamin C is a collagen booster and thus an important component of new antiaging products.

DOCTORS JOIN THE ANTIOXIDANT MOVEMENT

There is a movement in medicine as well to employ antioxidants as free radical scavengers. Free radicals are unpaired electrons that are due to a variety of causes including ultraviolet light, ozone, pollutants in the air we breathe, and environmental toxins. Free radicals, which are thought to destroy cells, have been linked to skin disease and premature aging as well as other medical problems. Antioxidants, in the form of ingestable vitamins and topical skin creams, may help obliterate free radicals. Well-known antioxidants include vitamin A, vitamin C, vitamin E, betacarotene, and bioflavonoids.

While hard research proving the benefits of antioxidants is

still lacking, most doctors are giving them increasing credence. Anecdotal evidence indicates that some doctors who are reluctant to recommend antioxidants to their patients—because of the lack of explicit supportive evidence—are nonetheless ingesting antioxidants themselves on a regular basis. Skepticism, on the other hand, exists as to whether any topical application of antioxidants is truly effective.

THE TOXIN THAT CAN SMOOTH YOUR FURROWED BROW

Also on the horizon is the surprising introduction of bo-tox, the botulism toxin, for cosmetic use. While still awaiting FDA approval, bo-tox appears to be both a safe and effective anti-wrinkle treatment. Many dermatologists, plastic surgeons, and ear, nose, and throat doctors are already injecting bo-tox into the furrowed brows of cosmetically challenged patients. The injection of bo-tox temporarily paralyzes the corrugator muscle, which is responsible for frown lines between the brows. For three to six months following the injection, a woman will be able to raise and lower her brows with nary a frown line showing.

LASERS: A VALUABLE TOOL IN DERMATOLOGY

Lasers are playing an increasingly important role in dermatology today. Scientists are experimenting with treating basal cell carcinomas and lymphomas with lasers in a procedure known as photodynamic therapy. Dermatologists have also expanded the use of lasers to include the removal of warts. The removal of tattoos through laser therapy is already a fast-growing trend in those who have suddenly outgrown these youthful symbols and now find them embarrassing. Lasers may someday even play a role in treating dilated veins and removing wrinkles and fine lines from skin.

GROWING NEW SKIN

One of the most remarkable new developments in dermatology has been the discovery that we can actually grow new skin. A small amount of your skin cells can be removed and grown in a culture medium until substantial new sheets of skin growth develop. Sheets of skin can then be used to cover skin defects. Once a process primarily for burn victims, today scientists are exploring the use of this new process in pigment disorders and even for cosmetic purposes.

NEW PERFORMANCE PRODUCTS: COSMECEUTICALS

Millions of dollars are being spent today on cosmeceuticals, "performance" or "treatment" products that hover somewhere between "beautifying" cosmetics and drugs that "affect the structure or function of the body." The first cosmeceutical to be approved by the FDA was minoxidil for hair growth. So far one alpha hydroxy acid or AHA has been approved for use on dry skin by the FDA, and it is likely that others will follow in the future.

Other skin care products that fall into the category of cosmeceuticals range from sunscreens to thigh creams that are applied to reduce the dimpled fat known as cellulite. While the merit of sunscreens is unquestioned and at least one study has shown that thigh creams can be helpful, some critics question the real value of thigh creams.

This only emphasizes the importance of doing your own homework and exercising good judgment in caring for your healthy skin.

APPENDIX I:

RESOURCES

ORGANIZATIONS AND PUBLICATIONS

The American Academy of Dermatology
930 North Meacham Road
Schaumburg, IL 60173-6016
(708) 330-0230

The American Academy of Dermatology provides a wealth of the most up-to-date and expert information on every aspect of skin care. Among its many pamphlets are "Skin Cancer: An Undeclared Epidemic," "The Sun and Your Skin," and "Skin Care Under the Sun."

American Academy of Facial, Plastic and Reconstructive Surgery
444 East Algonquin Road
Arlington Heights, IL 60065
(708) 228-9900
FAX (708) 228-9131

Brochures about facial plastic surgery are available. Representatives may also refer you to local plastic surgeons who are fellows of the American Academy of Facial, Plastic and Reconstructive Surgery (AAFPRS).

American Cancer Society
19 West 56th Street
New York, NY 10001
(212) 586-8700

The American Cancer Society is a good source of information on both skin cancer and how to quit smoking.

The American Heart Association
7320 Greenville Avenue
Dallas, TX 75231
(214) 750-5551

Local branches across the country offer information on the effects of smoking and how to quit.

American Lung Association
1740 Broadway
New York, NY 10019
(212) 315-8700

The American Lung Association offers advice on how to quit smoking on your own, and can also recommend helpful medical and psychological techniques.

American Society for Dermatologic Surgery
930 North Meacham Road
Schaumburg, IL 60173-6016
(708) 330-9830

Call for up-to-date information on dermatological surgical procedures.

American Society of Plastic and Reconstruction Surgeons
444 East Algonquin Road
Arlington Heights, IL 60065
(708) 228-9900

Call or write for information on all types of plastic surgery.

Center for Devices and Radiological Health
The Food and Drug Administration
5600 Fishers Lane
Rockville, MD 20857
(800) 638-2041

Free publications include "Out of the Bronzed Age," "Sunbathing Without Burning," and "PUVA's Double Whammy on Psoriasis."

Centers for Disease Control and Prevention
Division of Cancer Prevention and Control
4770 Buford Highway, NE K-64
Atlanta, GA 30341-3724
(404) 488-4751

Call or write for information about skin cancer.

Cleveland Clinic Foundation
Department of Dermatology and Department of Plastic Surgery
9500 Euclid Avenue
Cleveland, OH 44195-5001
(800) 223-2273

The Cleveland Clinic Foundation is a valuable source of information on a wide variety of skin problems.

Consumer Federation of America
1424 16th Street, NW
Suite 604
Washington, DC 20036
(202) 387-6121

Consumer Federation of America serves as the consumer representative on the Cosmetic Ingredient Review Panel (see below).

Consumer Information Center
P.O. Box 100
Pueblo, CO 81002

Write the Consumer Information Center for a list of free and low-priced pamphlets on a wide variety of subjects. Several, such as "Acne: Taming that Age-Old Adolescent Affliction," offer valuable tips on skin care.

Cosmetic Ingredient Review
1101 17th Street, NW
Suite 310
Washington, DC 20036-4702
(202) 331-0651

An educational resource about cosmetics and cosmetic ingredients.

Cosmetic Toiletry Fragrance Association
1101 17th Street, NW
Suite 300
Washington, DC 20036-4792

A good source of information about ingredients in fragrances, especially for allergic individuals.

Federal Trade Commission
Office of Consumer Education
Bureau of Consumer Protection
Washington, DC 20580
(202) 326-3650

Ask for their free publication on sunscreens.

The Food and Drug Administration
Office of Consumer Affairs
5600 Fishers Lane
Rockville, MD 20857
(301) 443-3170

The Food and Drug Administration offers free pamphlets such as "Contact Dermatitis: Solutions to Rash Mysteries."

National Alopecia Areata Foundation (NAAF)
710 C Street, Suite 11
P.O. Box 150760
San Rafael, CA 94915-0760
(415) 456-4666

Call or write for information on alopecia areata.

National Cancer Institute
Department of Health & Human Services
9000 Rockville Pike
Building 31, Room 10A24
Bethesda, MD 20892
(800) 4-CANCER

The National Cancer Institute will send you free publications and reprints of journal articles on skin and sunlight. Representatives can also give you the most up-to-date information on the treatment of skin cancer, including appropriate treatment of the various stages. The Physician's Data Query (PDQ) data base may be searched for any clinical studies of your disease. Free publications include "Skin Cancers: Basal and Squamous Cell Carcinomas," "What You Need to Know About Melanoma," and "What You Need to Know About Skin Cancer."

National Institute of Allergy and Infectious Diseases (NIAID)
Department of Health & Human Services
Building 31, Room 7A32
Bethesda, MD 20892
(301) 496-5717

Free publications are available on a wide variety of topics, including eczema, fungal infections such as athlete's foot, genital herpes and warts, hives, and poison ivy. The institute may also refer you to researchers and clinical studies.

National Institute of Arthritis and Musculoskeletal and Skin Diseases
(NIAMS)
Box AMS
9000 Rockville Pike
Bethesda, MD 20892
(301) 495-4484

NIAMS will send you free information on a wide variety of skin diseases, including acne, atopic dermatitis, and psoriasis. Publications often include reprints of recent medical journal articles. The institute can let you know of any clinical studies that may be studying your disease and looking for patients, as well as refer you to other organizations studying your particular problem.

National Institute of Dental Research
Department of Health & Human Services
Building 31, Room 2C35
Bethesda, MD 20892
(301) 496-4261

Call for a free pamphlet on "Fever Blisters and Canker Sores."

National Institute of Neurological Disorders and Stroke
Department of Health & Human Services
Building 31, Room 8A06
Bethesda, MD 20892
(800) 352-9424

This institute will send you free current publications on shingles (herpes zoster).

National Institute on Aging
Department of Health & Human Services
Building 31, Room 5C27
Bethesda, MD 20892
(800) 222-2225

The National Institute on Aging can send you free publications on skin and aging.

National Psoriasis Foundation
6443 S.W. Beaverton Highway
Suite 210
Portland, OR 97221
(503) 297-1545

Call or write for information about this common skin disorder.

National Rosacea Society
220 South Cook Street, Suite 201
Barrington, IL 60010

Write to this address for free information about rosacea, a skin disorder that may affect one out of twenty American adults.

National Sexually Transmitted Diseases Hotline
P.O. Box 13827
Research Triangle Park, NC 27707
(800) 227-8922

Call for free publications on sexually transmitted diseases, such as genital herpes and genital warts. Friendly and knowledgeable representatives on the hotline can answer your questions about how to protect yourself from as well as treat STDs.

National Vitiligo Foundation
P.O. Box 6337
Tyler, TX 75711
(903) 534-2925

Call for information and publications on this depigmentation condition.

Office of Cosmetics and Colors
The Food and Drug Administration
200 C Street, SW
Washington, DC 20204
(202) 205-4094

The FDA has a voluntary registration program for the producers of cosmetics; at present there is no mandatory program.

The office also has a data base in which they record complaints and allergic reactions to cosmetics. Call them to help you determine what steps to take if you experience an allergic reaction to a cosmetic product.

The Skin Cancer Foundation
245 Fifth Avenue
New York, NY 10016
(212) 725-5176

The foundation produces two free pamphlets for parents, "Sunproofing Your Baby" and "For Every Child Under the Sun: A Guide to Sensible Sun Protection." The book *Play It Safe in the Sun,* a helpful guide to both children and parents, is available for $12.90 (including shipping).

The Skin Phototrauma Foundation (SPF)
P.O. Box 6312
Parsippany, NJ 07054

Write to SPF for educational materials about the adverse effects of long-term sun exposure.

APPENDIX II: FURTHER READING

Elaine Brumberg. *Take Care of Your Skin.* New York: Harper & Row, 1989.

Nelson Lee Novick, M.D. *Super Skin.* New York: Clarkson Potter, 1988.

Linda Allen Schoen and Paul Lazar, M.D. *The Look You Like.* New York: Marcel Dekker, Inc., 1990.

Jan Willis. *Beautiful Again.* Santa Fe, NM: Health Press, 1994.

GLOSSARY

Acne: Medically known as *acne vulgaris,* an inflammatory skin condition of papules (solid red bumps), pustules (pus-filled bumps), whiteheads (closed comedones), and blackheads (open comedones) that most commonly appear on the face, neck, back, and chest when hair follicles become clogged with sebum (oil), keratin, bacteria or yeast; most common in adolescence when hormonal changes stimulate sebum production.

Actinic keratosis: A precancerous condition of small rough, red or brown, scaly patches on sun-exposed areas of skin.

Age spots: See Solar lentigines.

Alopecia: Baldness.

Alopecia areata: A condition of hair loss that affects approximately 2.5 million Americans, and is thought to be due to an underlying problem in the immune system.

Alpha hydroxy acids (AHAs): Naturally occurring acids in fruits and milk that are used topically to diminish fine wrinkles and dry skin.

Androgenetic alopecia: The most common form of baldness, which is caused by an excess of male hormones or androgens in susceptible individuals.

Androgens: Male hormones that are believed to be important in the development of acne, especially in both male and female teenagers, by enlarging oil glands and stimulating the production of pore-clogging sebum. An excess of androgens may also lead to androgenetic alopecia (baldness).

Angiomas: Common red-domed benign lesions on the trunk that may appear during pregnancy in genetically predisposed women; also become more numerous with age.

Antimicrobial: Germ-fighting.

Astringent: A liquid that may contain alcohol or other ingredients designed to cleanse oily residue from skin; astringents may have cooling, tingling, or tightening functions.

Athlete's foot: A fungal infection that manifests itself as sores between the toes or a scaling or blistering rash on the foot.

Atopy: The inherited predisposition to become allergic to substances such as pollen, ragweed, dust mites, molds, and animal scales or droppings.

Basal cell carcinoma: The most common form of skin cancer, originating in the basal cells of the epidermis. A slow-growing cancer that seldom spreads and accounts for about 90 percent of all skin cancers in the United States.

Basal cells: Small, round cells in the lower part of the epidermis.

Basement membrane: The connection between the dermis and the epidermis: a series of fingerlike projections called papillae that weave the two layers together. (Also called the dermal/epidermal junction.)

Benign: Not cancerous.

Biopsy: The removal of a sample of tissue to determine under a microscope whether or not cancer cells are present.

Blackheads: Open comedones typical of acne; colored black because of melanin.

Blisters: Small swellings of the skin filled with watery matter; caused by friction.

Boils: Tender, red, inflamed lesions, medically known as furuncles.

Broad spectrum sunscreen: A sunscreen that filters out both UVB and UVA rays. (See also Sunscreen.)

Bunions: Inflammations of the skin and bone swelling at the base of the big toe.

Calluses: Hardened or thickened areas of skin.

Cancer: A group of diseases in which cells become abnormal, dividing too often and without regard to control or order.

Carcinogen: Any substance that causes cancer.

Carcinoma: A cancer that begins in the cells that line or cover an organ.

Cellulite: Dimpled skin caused by compartmentalization of fat cells.

Chemical peel: A nonsurgical procedure in which acid is used to resurface skin, thus eliminating fine wrinkles, age spots, and actinic keratoses.

Clinical trials: Research studies with patients in which doctors study new treatments for skin cancer and other diseases.

Collagen: A substance in the dermis layer of the skin that prevents skin from tearing; imparts thickness and strength to skin.

Collagen injection: A nonsurgical procedure in which purified bovine collagen is injected into wrinkles to make them temporarily disappear.

Comedones: Acne lesions that may be open (blackheads) or closed (whiteheads) and occur when follicles become clogged with sebum, dead skin cells, and bacteria.

Corns: Horny and often painful thickenings of the skin, most common on toes, and caused by friction or compression.

Corticosteroids: Anti-inflammatory drugs used to treat a wide range of dermatological conditions, such as eczema and psoriasis.

Cosmeceuticals: Drugs that are used for cosmetic purposes—that is, for enhancing appearance.

Cryosurgery: Also known as cryotherapy, a freezing technique using liquid nitrogen which blisters off superficial tumors and cancers.

Curettage: A procedure most often used to treat basal cell carcinoma, in which cancer is scooped out with a sharp, spoon-shaped instrument called a curette.

Curette: An instrument with a sharp, spoon-shaped end used in curettage; used to scrape skin.

Cutaneous: Related to the skin.

Cysts: Small closed sacs that contain microorganisms, keratin, cellular debris, and oil gland secretions; milia and follicular cysts are two common forms.

Dandruff: The shedding of dead skin cells from the scalp.

Dermabrasion: A nonsurgical procedure in which a hand-held, high-speed rotary wheel is used to remove the top layer of skin in order to eliminate imperfections such as scars and deep wrinkles.

Dermatitis: Inflammation of the skin; often used synonymously with *eczema,* which refers more specifically to noninfectious skin rashes.

Dermatologist: A doctor who specializes in diseases of the skin.

Dermis: The inner layer of the skin.

Dysplastic nevi: Moles that appear different from normal moles due to asymmetry, border irregularity, a lack of uniform color, or a large diameter.

Eczema: Often used as a synonym for *dermatitis,* an umbrella term referring to a wide range of skin rashes; eczema is not caused by germs and therefore is not contagious.

Elastin: A substance in the dermis layer of the skin that makes skin resilient.

Electrodesiccation: A procedure in which electric current is applied to the affected area to control bleeding and destroy any remaining cancer cells.

Electrosurgery: A generic term used for various forms of electrical destruction of a lesion.

Epidermis: The outer layer of the skin.

Exfoliator: Exfoliators slough off the surface layer of dead skin cells; exfoliating scrubs may be used in the treatment of acne or to give skin a fresher and more youthful appearance.

Fat injection: A nonsurgical procedure in which a person's own fat is removed from his or her buttocks or thigh and injected into wrinkles to smooth and eliminate them.

Flat warts: Smooth, velvety, and regularly shaped warts caused by the papilloma virus.

Fluorouracil: An anticancer drug used in the topical chemotherapy of skin cancer.

Follicles: Pores; openings or sacs in the dermis from which hair grows.

Folliculitis: Inflammation of the hair follicles, characterized by many small red bumps (papules) or pus bumps (pustules) in the hair follicle openings where the hair meets the skin.

Freckles: Small benign brown spots that commonly appear on the face and arms; often a sign of sun damage.

Furuncles: Tender, red, inflamed lesions commonly known as boils.

Genital herpes: A viral skin infection characterized by sores in the genital area; spread through intimate contact.

Genital warts: Warts in the genital region caused by the human papilloma virus; spread through intimate contact.

Hemorrhoids: Varicose veins in the anal area.

Herpes zoster: A cluster of blisters on a reddish base that results from reactivation of the chicken pox virus many years after the original outbreak of chicken pox; the symptoms range from mild to severe. (Also called *shingles*.)

Hyperhidrosis: Excessive sweating to an unusual degree.

Hyperpigmentation: The darkening of certain skin areas that sometimes takes place during pregnancy due to heightened hormonal stimulation.

Hypopigmentation: The lightening or depigmentation of skin patches.

Jogger's nipples: Inflamed, itchy and sensitive skin of nipples due to trauma, usually rubbing of a T-shirt or bra while engaged in athletic activity.

Impetigo: The most common bacterial skin infection, which is very contagious and frequently affects children.

Kaposi's sarcoma: A type of blood vessel cancer that develops on the skin of people who have a weakened immune system; frequently the first presenting sign of HIV infection.

Keloids: Hard scars; fleshy lesions caused by overgrown scar tissue due to severe acne, injury, burns, or surgery.

Keratin: A tightly compacted protein found in your skin, hair, and nails that, to varying degrees, helps them act as protective barriers between you and the outside world.

Liposuction: A surgical procedure for the removal of unwanted or excess fat cells from the body.

Lymphatic system: The system of organs, tissues, and tubes that produces, stores, and carries body liquid. The human lymph system acts as a barrier against cancer; once cancer has metastasized to the lymph glands, the prognosis is poor.

Macules: Nonelevated skin spots characteristic of eczema; color ranges from red to black.

Malignant: Cancerous.

Mast cells: Cells in the skin that release histamine in response to contact with an allergen, causing symptoms such as itching and inflammation.

Melanin: The pigment that gives our skin its color.

Melanocytes: Cells in the skin that contain and produce melanin.

Melanoma: The most serious type of skin cancer; abnormal proliferation of melanocytes, which become a cancer and quickly metastasize; can be fatal.

Melasma: "The mask of pregnancy," or a darkening of pigmentation on facial skin during pregnancy due to some combination of hormonal changes, overexposure to the sun, and genetic factors.

Metastasis: The spread of cancer.

Minoxidil: The only topical treatment currently approved by the Food and Drug Administration (FDA) for the treatment of androgenetic alopecia (hereditary hair loss); sold under the brand name Rogaine.

Mohs' technique: A highly specialized type of surgery in which a cancer is removed one thin layer at a time. Used in hard-to-treat, recurrent nonmelanoma skin cancers. Cancer is removed in layers and reviewed by dermatologist to ensure that entire cancer is removed.

Mole: A cluster of melanocytes that appears as a dark spot on the skin.

Mycosis fungoides: Also known as T-cell lymphoma, a cancer of the immune system that may first appear on the skin and has recently been associated with HIV.

Nevus (pigmented): A mole, or cluster of melanocytes that appears as a dark spot on the skin.

Noncomedogenic: Does not clog pores.

Nonmelanoma skin cancer: Basal cell and squamous cell carcinoma are often jointly referred to as nonmelanoma skin cancer in order to distinguish them from far more serious malignant melanoma.

PABA: Para-aminobenzoic acid, a common ingredient in sunscreens; women with sensitive or allergy-prone skin should choose PABA-free products.

Papillae: Fingerlike projections of the dermis that interlace with overlying epidermis as the basement membrane; ball and glove connection that binds the two layers.

Papules: Small bumps that may be red, white, or flesh-colored.

Pathologist: A doctor who identifies diseases by studying cells under a microscope; a dermatological pathologist specializes in skin pathology.

Photoaging: Also known as photodamage and phototrauma, damage to the skin due to cumulative exposure to the sun. Much of the wrinkling, lines, and brown spots that used to be considered part of natural chronological aging are now attributed to ultraviolet exposure from sunlight or artificial sources, such as tanning booths and sunlamps.

Pigment: A substance that gives color to tissue.

Pityriasis rosea: A benign skin rash that usually begins with a single pink patch on the chest or back and then spreads.

Pores: Tiny openings in the skin's surface; also known as hair follicles.

Precancerous: A condition that may develop into cancer.

Prognosis: The probable outcome of a disease.

Pruritus: Itching.

Psoriasis: A chronic, noncontagious skin disease characterized by red, scaly patches that may itch or sting; although there are many treatments for psoriasis, at present there is no cure for the condition.

Pustules: Pus bumps characteristic of many skin rashes, such as acne and impetigo.

Pyodermas: Bacterial infections of the skin.

Radiation therapy: A method in which high-energy rays are used to kill cancer cells; may be used to treat nonmelanoma skin cancers, particularly in the elderly.

Retin-A: A topical drug, available by prescription only, that was originally designed and is still used to fight acne; in 1988 researchers suggested that Retin-A could reverse the effects of photoaging, and today Retin-A is one of the most popular antiaging medications.

Rhinophyma: A puffy, swollen red nose associated with rosacea in men.

Rosacea: A skin disease characterized by varying degrees of facial redness and thin red lines due to the enlargement and dilation of blood vessels beneath the skin's surface; as redness progresses, pimples may also appear, which has often led to rosacea being mislabeled as acne.

Seborrhea: A combination of increased oil (sebum) and scaling off of dead skin cells from the scalp.

Seborrheic dermatitis: The normal flaking of seborrhea accompanied by redness, itching, and greasy scales or crusts most commonly found on the scalp, eyebrows, eyelids, and face; thought to be caused by the yeast pityrosporon orbiculare.

Sebum: An oily substance produced in the dermis that keeps the skin from drying out.

Shingles: See Herpes zoster.

Skin tags: Harmless, flesh-colored skin that hangs on fine stalks; also known by their dermatological names, papillomas and acrochordon.

Smoker's face: A condition of pale and sallow color along with wrinkles radiating from the eyes and chin that is due to chronic smoking.

Solar lentigines: The dermatological term for age or liver spots, these are flat, brown macules that may appear on the face, hands, back, and feet; they are caused by cumulative exposure to the sun.

Spider veins: Dilated or broken blood vessels near the surface of the skin; in medical terminology, telangiectasias.

Squamous cell carcinoma: The second most common form of skin cancer, originating in the squamous cells of the epidermis.

Squamous cells: Flat cells that make up most of the epidermis.

Stratum corneum: The surface scales of your skin or top layer of your epidermis.

Subcutaneous tissue: The bottom layer of skin, composed mostly of fat, that provides valuable insulation and storage for nutrients and drugs.

Sun Protection Factor (SPF): A scale that rates the level of protection that sunscreens provide from the UVB rays of the sun. The American Academy of Dermatology recommends using a broad spectrum sunscreen with an SPF of 15 or higher.

Sunblock: A substance that protects your skin from the harmful rays of the sun by *reflecting* ultraviolet rays. Active ingredients include titanium dioxide and zinc oxide; because sunblocks are not absorbed by the skin, in the past they tended to be opaque and visible.

Today's formulas contain absorbers that make them more attractive to use.

Sunscreen: A substance that protects your skin from the harmful rays of the sun by *absorbing* ultraviolet rays. Formerly, sunscreens offered protection only against UVB rays; today's broad spectrum sunscreens also offer protection from UVA rays.

Suntan lotion: A lotion designed to moisturize the skin and permit tanning. Offers little or no sun protection.

Telangiectasias: The medical term for spider veins or superficial, broken blood vessels.

Topical chemotherapy: The application to a precancerous or skin cancer growth of the anticancer drug 5-fluorouracil (5-U) as a cream or solution on a daily basis for several weeks. Used to treat actinic keratoses and some superficial basal cell and squamous cell carcinomas.

Tumor: An abnormal mass or overgrowth of tissue that may be benign or cancerous.

Ultraviolet radiation: Energy given off by the sun that can damage your skin and lead to skin cancer. (Also see UVA and UVB radiation.)

UVA radiation: Long wavelengths emitted by the sun. UVA rays take longer than those of UVB to produce a burn, but also penetrate deeper into your skin and may damage collagen, the elastic substance that keeps skin young and firm. More recently, scientists have begun to associate UVA rays with skin damage that may lead to melanoma, photoaging, and nonmelanoma skin cancer.

UVB radiation: Short wavelengths emitted by the sun that have long been associated with sun damage and skin cancer. Most intense between the hours of 10 A.M. and 3 P.M. standard time, in the summer months, and in climates close to and south of the equator.

Varicose veins: Abnormally or irregularly swollen veins, especially in the legs.

Vesicles: Small blisters in the skin that contain clear liquid.

Vitiligo: A condition of depigmented skin patches; a type of hypopigmentation.

Whiteheads: Closed comedones typical of acne; also known as milia or cysts.

INDEX

ABOUT THE AUTHORS

WILMA F. BERGFELD, M.D., F.A.C.P., is head of Clinical Research in the Department of Dermatology and head of Dermatopathology in the Department of Pathology at The Cleveland Clinic Foundation in Cleveland, Ohio. She attended Temple University Medical School and completed her internship and residency at The Cleveland Clinic Foundation. Dr. Bergfeld has authored over 400 peer-reviewed publications. She is a board certified dermatologist and dermatopathologist and a recent past president of a number of dermatologic and medical societies, including the American Academy of Dermatology and the Women's Dermatologic Society. Dr. Bergfeld is the current chairwoman of the FDA Dermatology Advisory Committee and the chairwoman of the Cosmetic Ingredient Review expert panel. She lives in Cleveland, Ohio.

SHELAGH RYAN MASLINE is a writer and editor who specializes in health-related subjects. She has contributed to more than a dozen titles, and most recently has coauthored *Living with Asthma* and *Healing Herbal Remedies*. She lives in New York City.